Enhancing Nurses' and Midwives' Competence in Providing Spiritual Care

Wilfred McSherry • Adam Boughey

Josephine Attard

Editors

Enhancing Nurses' and Midwives' Competence in Providing Spiritual Care

Through Innovative Education and Compassionate Care

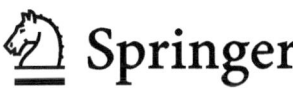 Springer

11 *Editors*
Wilfred McSherry
Department of Nursing, School of Health
and Social Care
Staffordshire University
Stoke-On-Trent
UK

Adam Boughey
Department of Nursing, School of Health
and Social Care
Staffordshire University
Stoke-On-Trent
UK

Josephine Attard
Faculty of Health Sciences
University of Malta
Msida
Malta

12 ISBN 978-3-030-65887-8   ISBN 978-3-030-65888-5   (eBook)
13 https://doi.org/10.1007/978-3-030-65888-5

14 © Springer Nature Switzerland AG 2021
15 This work is subject to copyright. All rights are reserved by the Publisher, whether the whole or part of
16 the material is concerned, specifically the rights of translation, reprinting, reuse of illustrations, recitation,
17 broadcasting, reproduction on microfilms or in any other physical way, and transmission or information
18 storage and retrieval, electronic adaptation, computer software, or by similar or dissimilar methodology
19 now known or hereafter developed.
20 The use of general descriptive names, registered names, trademarks, service marks, etc. in this publication
21 does not imply, even in the absence of a specific statement, that such names are exempt from the relevant
22 protective laws and regulations and therefore free for general use.
23 The publisher, the authors and the editors are safe to assume that the advice and information in this book
24 are believed to be true and accurate at the date of publication. Neither the publisher nor the authors or the
25 editors give a warranty, expressed or implied, with respect to the material contained herein or for any
26 errors or omissions that may have been made. The publisher remains neutral with regard to jurisdictional
27 claims in published maps and institutional affiliations.

28 This Springer imprint is published by the registered company Springer Nature Switzerland AG
29 The registered company address is: Gewerbestrasse 11, 6330 Cham, Switzerland

Foreword

In a secular society like the UK there appears to be a reticence by some nurses and
midwives to talk to patients/clients about their beliefs, the importance of religious
faith and their spiritual well-being as part of the package of care provided to them.
This reticence could stem from an anxiety they may offend the person by saying the
wrong thing, because they feel ill-equipped to have meaningful conversations or
they are unaware they need to provide this aspect of care. The end result of this is
that many vulnerable and sick people cannot access the spiritual support they need
at a time when they need it most.

I have been a nurse for just over 40 years, and it has been a privilege to have supported many sick, frail and vulnerable people during this time. I have experienced
joy and sorrow when being with individuals and their families through all kinds of
episodes of care, from the joy of birth to the sorrow of death. From my personal
experiences, I have learnt that to care effectively for a person you must develop an
understanding not just of the person's physical, emotional and social needs but also
what gives meaning to that person's life. For some people they will find meaning
through religious beliefs and will take comfort from the associated religious rituals
that accompany that faith; for others, personal beliefs and values that guide the way
they live their lives and treat others enable them to give meaning to their lives and
experiences. I have observed that how we interact with the world and the meaning
we attribute to things change with time and life events, such as becoming a parent,
developing a life-limiting disease or losing a loved one. How we deal with the challenge's life throws at us is heavily coloured by our beliefs, and I have seen great
differences in the way people react to illness, injury or a failing in their health and
physical abilities. Providing nursing or midwifery care without acknowledging the
spiritual aspect of person's life ultimately denies something fundamental about the
people for whom we provide care.

Health and social care services and the models of care provided by professionals
are constantly evolving. This evolution reflects the changing expectations and needs
of our population as well as embracing advances in medicines and technology.
However, while services and care pathways change over time, one thing that should

not change is positioning the individual at the centre of care decisions. In recent
years, the importance of co-producing care and treatment plans with the people
receiving care has risen in prominence. Health professionals must take into account
the recipient's beliefs, expectations, fears and unique living arrangements when
making care plans. Part of any undergraduate nursing and midwifery education programme must therefore concentrate on what person-centred holistic care means and
this must include spiritual care as a facet. While academics and the professional
regulator accept the need to include aspects of belief, faith and cultural diversity in
any education programme, the question remains however about how best to deliver
such material.

When I heard about the planned European research project to develop awareness
and competency in nurses and midwives to support the spiritual needs of people
receiving health and social care, I was determined that Wales would contribute. A
significant part of my portfolio in Welsh Government is to ensure a safe, positive
patient experience, and as part of this work, Welsh Government has set standards for
the spiritual care of people receiving healthcare. However, I have always been concerned about how the workforce, particularly the nursing and midwifery professionals who provide the majority of care, were interpreting and implementing these
standards and whether they had the skill set to do this aspect of care well. Having
said that, there are pockets of excellence in Wales and I was pleased that some of
these experts were able to contribute to the project. I would like to take this opportunity to express my thanks to them for their willingness to travel and give of their
personal time to take part in this project.

The 'Enhancing Nurses' and Midwives' Competence in Providing Spiritual Care
through Innovative Education and Compassionate Care' (EPICC) European project
provided the space for international experts to consider how best to promote awareness and provide skills in offering spiritual care. The products from this project
include: a spiritual care education standard; a matrix diagram showing the cultural,
social and political environment in which spiritual care competency develops with
supporting narrative; and core spiritual care competencies for undergraduate nursing and midwifery students. These products not only advise on good practice for
teaching and assessment but also help guide student selection decisions.

In this book, the findings from this 3-year project (2016–2019), conducted with
engagement from over 49 participants (nursing and midwifery educators, in addition to key stakeholders and students) from 21 European countries, are described in
detail. Most of the chapters were written/coordinated by one of the EPICC strategic
partners who led the EPICC project and co-authored by five of the EPICC participants (those experts who participated in the EPICC project). The chapters set out
informed discussion points and are presented in an engaging and interactive way to
help build confidence and understanding in the reader. It means that rather than
being a typical textbook, this book becomes a resource guide for educators as well
as students.

One of the most important steps any student can take on their journey to be a
well-rounded and competent professional is to begin understanding himself or herself. Some of the concepts in this book will challenge the reader to examine their

personal beliefs and prejudices; what role faith and beliefs have in everyday life; 106
and explore some of the existential challenges we all face: for example, hope and 107
despair, questions about identity, and the meaning of life itself. Understanding how 108
our upbringing and the cultural and political environment in which we exist all have 109
a part to play in how we see the world around us. Recognising that the recipients of 110
our care may well have had very different experiences to us and therefore hold dif- 111
ferent values and beliefs is essential. 112

The work of a nurse or midwife can be challenging, and clinical environments 113
can be busy demanding places in which to work, and it can be all too easy to rush 114
from one job to another and forget about the person receiving care. For them it is 115
anything but routine and is uniquely stressful. The content of this book reminds the 116
reader that even in a busy clinical environment it is essential to make time to connect 117
with the human being receiving care and have meaningful conversations with that 118
person about what matters to them. This is the art of caring: to see past the tasks and 119
see the person beneath. 120

I hope you enjoy reading and interacting with the material presented in this book. 121

April 2020 Jean White 122
Health and Social Services Group 123
Welsh Government 124
Wales, UK 125

Contents

288 289 290 291 292 293 294 295 296 297 298 299 300 301 302 303 304 305 306 307 308 309 310 311 312 313 314 315 316 317 318 319 320

Chapter 1
The EPICC Project: Inception, Origins and Outputs

Wilfred McSherry, Adam Boughey, and Josephine Attard

Learning Objectives

This chapter will:

1. Provide a summary of the EPICC project and why this was necessary to advance nursing and midwifery, practice, research and education.
2. Introduce, the key outputs arising from the EPICC project, demonstrating how these can be used within nursing and midwifery education.
3. Offer an overview of the book, discussing the contribution this will make to nursing and midwifery practice, research and education.

1.1 Introduction

The EPICC project has laid the foundations to help reduce the gap and disconnect between professional regulatory bodies' statements and aspirations for high-quality spiritual care and actual practice. Recent definitions of spirituality suggest that

W. McSherry (✉)
Department of Nursing, School of Health and Social Care, University Hospitals of North Midlands NHS Trust, Staffordshire University, Stoke-on-Trent, Staffordshire, England, UK

VID University College, Bergen/Oslo, Norway
e-mail: w.mcsherry@staffs.ac.uk

A. Boughey
Department of Nursing, School of Health and Social Care, Staffordshire University, Stoke-on-Trent, Staffordshire, England, UK
e-mail: adam.boughey@staffs.ac.uk

J. Attard
University of Malta, Msida, Malta
e-mail: josephine.attard@um.edu.mt

© Springer Nature Switzerland AG 2021
W. McSherry et al. (eds.), *Enhancing Nurses' and Midwives' Competence in Providing Spiritual Care*, https://doi.org/10.1007/978-3-030-65888-5_1

spirituality is multidimensional and unique to every person [1]. It is broader than religious beliefs and is about meaning in life, connection to self, others and/or higher power or nature [2]. It provides ways to transcend everyday living and suffering [3]. Murgia et al. ([4], p. 14) conclude a recent concept analysis of spirituality in nursing by stating:

> To this end, nurses need sound theoretical foundations to recognise the different spiritual meanings of important periods of life for patients as birth, death and suffering, and link them to ethical issues in the practice of care.

This recommendation affirms that the concept of spirituality is important at all key life events including birth emphasising the fundamental role this dimension also plays in midwifery practice. The importance of ensuring that nurses and midwives have a 'sound theoretical' knowledge base was one of the major aspirations of the EPICC project.

The EPICC objectives were to:

1. Develop a sustainable network of educators in nursing/midwifery in Europe to share experiences on person-centred and compassionate healthcare working according to European standards.
2. Disseminate knowledge amongst stakeholders (policymakers, regulatory bodies and educational bodies) across Europe to enable the EPICC Gold Standard Matrix to be incorporated into ongoing nursing/midwifery education.

1.2   Why EPICC Was Needed?

The spiritual dimension of healthcare over the course of several decades has been a source of contention and viewed with a degree of scepticism. Part of the reason for this may stem from the subjectivity of the concept and the misconceptions associated with the meaning and interpretation of this word. However, in recent times, there has been a growing realisation of the importance and significance of this dimension for the health and well-being of individuals with many governments now valuing the contribution this makes to the health of their citizens [5], especially those facing key life events such as birth, illness and/or death [6–10]. There is also an emerging evidence base that reinforces the potential benefits to general health, well-being, quality of life and coping with conditions such as anxiety/depression [11–13].

It has been suggested that spiritual care is that care which responds to people's personal, religious and spiritual beliefs and needs emphasising how this may be important to accessing healthcare [14–17]. This means this dimension of care must be taken seriously by those providing services [18–20] but is often overlooked [14, 16, 21]. Despite a recognition of the importance of this dimension to the delivery of

care within the UK, there have been an increasing number of reports that shed light 46
on significant failings in the quality and standards of care [22–27]. Reviewing the 47
failings suggests that care was lacking in compassion, meaning individuals were not 48
treated with dignity and respect. These attributes [dignity and respect] have been 49
shown to be synonymous with spirituality [28–30]. Sir Robert Francis, who led the 50
2013 Public Inquiry into The Mid Staffordshire NHS Foundation Trust, stated high- 51
quality care 'puts the patient first', ensuring that they are the focal point for the 52
provision of all care, services and treatments. 53

A consequence of not focusing and building services around the needs of the 54
'person' whether this be the patient, carer or staff is that they are at risk of fostering 55
cultures, values, attitudes and behaviours that may lead to dignity violations since 56
there is a failure to recognise the humanity and dignity of each person. As stated, the 57
European Commission [5] highlights the need for all those involved in the caring 58
professions to be prepared to support the spiritual, religious and cultural needs of 59
people. This is also reflected and endorsed by some of the nursing and midwifery 60
regulatory and educational bodies who stress the importance of providing holistic 61
and person-centred care especially at the point of registration [31–34]. Despite this 62
recognition within the nursing and midwifery professions, there is still a great deal 63
of uncertainty about what spirituality is and how to provide spiritual care [35]. The 64
notion of spirituality and spiritual care is explored in Chap. 2. 65

The specific focus and context of this chapter, and indeed the work of the EPICC 66
project, were on developments within Europe involving nursing and midwifery. The 67
EPICC project sought to address several gaps identified (Table 1.1) in the existing 68
knowledge base and practice of spiritual care. 69

Table 1.1 Gaps in nurse/midwifery spiritual care education[a]   t1.1

1.	It was not clear what spiritual care competency looked like or how it might be assessed; there were no spiritual care competencies
2.	It was unclear how learners might acquire spiritual caring skills
3.	Spiritual care teaching within undergraduate nurse/midwifery education programmes was inconsistent, and in some places non-existent [36, 37]
4.	Practising nurses/midwives reported over several decades that they felt inadequately prepared for spiritual care and in need of further education [35, 38, 39]
5.	Whilst some educational materials were available for practising nurses/midwives (e.g., Royal College of Nursing (RCN) [35], online educational resources), the evidence on which to base them was scant, and no educational materials were publicly available for pre-registration nurses/midwives

t1.2
t1.3
t1.4
t1.5
t1.6
t1.7
t1.8
t1.9
t1.10
t1.11
t1.12

[a]Table 1.1 reproduced with kind permission from Taylor and Francis from the article McSherry W, t1.13
Ross L, Attard J, van Leeuwen R, Giske T, Kleiven T, Boughey A, and the EPICC Network (2020) t1.14
Preparing undergraduate nurses and midwives for spiritual care: Some developments in European t1.15
education over the last decade Journal for the Study of Spirituality 10(1) 55–71 doi: https://doi. t1.16
org/10.1080/20440243.2020.1726053 t1.17

1.3   Origins and Organisation of the EPICC Project

1.3.1   Origins

The publication of this book detailing the inception, origins and achievements of the EPICC project should not be viewed as a single point in time. The completion of this book denotes a significant milestone for many of the contributors. Since this work builds on many of the authors' pioneering and seminal research spanning several decades. This book is essentially not the culmination of a programme of work but the continuation of a journey seeking the advancement of spiritual care education, research and practice. This journey commenced many decades earlier with passionate individuals who held a shared vision of ensuring that our nursing and midwifery professions, indeed the whole of healthcare, were truly person-centred and holistic.

1.3.2   European Spirituality Research Network for Nursing and Midwifery

A landmark meeting took place at Staffordshire University on 20 August 2009, where the decision was taken to set up an informal network titled 'European Spirituality Research Network for Nursing and Midwifery'. The aim of this network was to:

- *Advance collaborative research into spirituality within nursing and midwifery across Europe and beyond.*

And the objective was:

- *Through scholarly activity and collaborative research explore the relevance of spirituality within nursing and midwifery practice and education.*

At this inaugural meeting, one of the actions was for the network to undertake an international study provisionally titled 'Cross-cultural investigation of student nurses' perceptions of spirituality and preparedness to deliver spiritual care'.

This research was built on an earlier work undertaken by [40] that explored the ethics of teaching spirituality to undergraduate student nurses. This research involved two phases:

1. **Pilot study** [41, 42] which was undertaken during 2010. The pilot involved a cross-sectional study of 531 pre-registration nursing/midwifery students from six universities in four European countries (Wales, Norway, Netherlands, and Malta). The main findings from this pilot phase were:

    (a) Students held a broad view of spirituality (measured by the Spirituality & 103
        Spiritual Care Rating Scale [SSCRS]; [43]). 104
    (b) Students considered themselves to be more competent than not in spiritual 105
        care (measured by Spiritual Care Competency Scale [SCCS]; [44]) at the 106
        start of their studies. 107

2. **The main study** [45] was conducted between 2011 and 2016, comprising a lon- 108
   gitudinal prospective follow-on study of 2193 (dropping to 595) students from 109
   21 universities in eight European countries. The results: 110

    (a) Confirmed the findings from the pilot study; personal spirituality of the stu- 111
        dent (high spirituality scores preferable [SAIL $p < 0.01$; JAREL $p < 0.01$) 112
        and perception of spirituality (holding a broad view preferable, SSCRS 113
        $p < 0.01$) positively correlated with perceived spiritual care compe- 114
        tency (SCC). 115
    (b) SCC developed significantly over the duration of the course of study 116
        ($p < 0.01$), which students attributed to caring for patients in clinical prac- 117
        tice, personal life events and teaching/discussion in university and with 118
        other students. 119

   The findings from these two ground-breaking studies provided clear evidence 120
and direction for nursing and midwifery educators. They highlighted what should be 121
taught in programmes of education, and importantly, they offered insights into what 122
strategies can help students to become competent in the delivery of spiritual care. 123

1.3.2.1   A Significant Milestone for Spiritual Care Competencies 124
in Nursing and Midwifery 125

The whole area of competency development in nursing and midwifery practice has 126
been the subject of much debate with several of the leading scholars in this area 127
participating in the EPICC project. The success of the EPICC project hinged on the 128
fact that the project was not starting with a 'blank canvas' as it built on existing 129
work. One of the foundational works was a PhD study conducted by Dr. Josephine 130
Attard undertaken between 2011 and 2015. This PhD study developed the first spiri- 131
tual care competency framework for pre-registration nurses/midwives. The research 132
involved an in-depth review of the international literature, stakeholder focus groups 133
and modified Delphi method. The outcome of this body of work was the construc- 134
tion of an educational framework that comprised of 54 items arranged in 7 domains: 135
knowledge in spiritual care; self-awareness and the use of self; communication and 136
interpersonal skills; ethical and legal issues; quality assurance in spiritual care; 137
assessment and implementation of spiritual care; informatics in spiritual care [46]. 138
This pioneering and unique framework was used as the starting point in the develop- 139
ment of the EPICC Spiritual Care Education Standard. 140

1.3.3 Organisation and Delivery of EPICC

Most of the founding members of the European Spirituality Research Network for Nursing and Midwifery were involved in the development of the EPICC funding application. After three successive attempts, the Network was finally awarded funding. This was through the Erasmus+ Key Action 2 Strategic Partnerships for Higher Education funding stream. The funding was awarded by the United Kingdom (UK) National Agency to conduct the project titled: 'Enhancing Nurses Competence in Providing Spiritual Care through Innovative Education and Compassionate Care (EPICC)'.[1]

1.3.3.1 EPICC Strategic Partners and EPICC Project Manager

The EPICC Strategic Partners are pioneers in this area of nursing and midwifery education and practice both within their own institutions, countries and internationally. They are acknowledged as leading experts in this field and have consistently championed this fundamental dimension of people's lives. EPICC can be considered innovative because it united a disparate field of nursing and midwifery education, research and practice. The EPICC Strategic Partners have collaborated in this area for over 20 years. This collaboration has resulted in several pioneering scholarly outputs including the publication of articles, books/chapters, and symposium presentations at international conferences and the development of spiritual care guidance.

The EPICC project brought together established experts, allowing them to share their expertise and knowledge with other less-experienced colleagues from some of the underrepresented countries in Europe, for example Croatia, Turkey and Ukraine. Throughout the course of the project, they provided mentorship, supervision and coaching to develop participants' knowledge, skills and expertise in this neglected aspect of nursing and midwifery education.

All the EPICC Strategic Partners were, and still are, involved in the education and continuing professional development of nurses and midwives at undergraduate and postgraduate levels, and all have doctorates in spiritual aspects of nursing and midwifery. Collectively, they have a vast array of skills and competence in educational and research methods. Some also have a clinical element to their roles which enables excellent integration of theory and practice.

Each EPICC Strategic Partner made a unique contribution to the implementation and administration of the project, as outlined below and in Table 1.4:

---

[1] The Grant Agreement Number was: 2016–1-UK01-KA203–024467) and the total grant awarded: €242,093.

- Professor Wilfred McSherry assumed overall leadership for the programme of work, working with colleagues at Staffordshire University, such as Isobel Walker, Tom Ward, and Mandy Welch. The daily management and delivery of the project was undertaken by Dr. Adam Boughey, who was employed by Staffordshire University as the EPICC Project Manager.
- Professor Linda Ross (nee Waugh) was involved in the development of 'intellectual output 1'[2] and the coordination of the second 'Multiplier event'.[3]
- Professor Tove Giske was involved in the development, establishment and sustainability of the EPICC Network. She was also involved in the administration and coordination of the EPICC project along with Professor McSherry.
- Professor René van Leeuwen coordinated intellectual output 2, along with the first learning/teaching/training activities (LTTAs) (C1) at Viaa Christian University.
- Professor Tormod Kleiven ensured the entire EPICC programme was informed by the voice of nurses, students and representatives from patient/public groups and professional regulatory bodies, which was an integral aspect of intellectual output 1.
- Professor Donia Baldacchino was involved in the development of the application for the funding of EPICC. Sadly, just after being notified of the successful outcome of the award, Professor Baldacchino was diagnosed with terminal cancer and died on 30 March 2017. We dedicate the entire project in her memory. Fortunately, for the EPICC project, Dr. Josephine Attard, one of Prof Baldacchino's PhD students at that time, was able to take on the responsibility for leading intellectual output 3 and was coordinator of the second learning/teaching/training activities (LTTAs) (C2) at the University of Malta.

  It should be highlighted that Professor Baldacchino's legacy continues in the research, publications and conference presentations that she presented over several decades but most importantly in the students and healthcare professionals she has inspired to engage with spiritual care.

The six EPICC Strategic Partners were responsible for achieving all the intellectual outputs, organising the four project events (two learning/teaching/training activities and two multiplier events). This group provided intense peer-support, mentorship, supervision to the EPICC Participants, monitoring progress and ensuring milestones were achieved. Professor McSherry, as the lead Strategic Partner, obtained the appropriate ethical approval for the project. This was to ensure that all the project intellectual outputs could be used to inform reports, publications and other dissemination activities.

---

[2] '"Intellectual output" is an activity that results in tangible and meaningful outcomes, such as publications and course materials' [46].

[3] '"Multiplier event" is an event that is organised to share the intellectual output of a project with a wider audience' [46].

1.4 Participating Groups

The EPICC project involved three key groups: 6 EPICC Strategic Partners (outlined above); 31 EPICC Participants (http://blogs.staffs.ac.uk/epicc/epicc-participants/), who were nursing/midwifery educators from across Europe; and 18 EPICC Participants+, who were key stakeholders, students, members of the public, professional bodies and patient groups. Collectively, these three groups comprised sides of the 'EPICC Triangle' (Fig. 1.1).

The involvement of these three groups ensured that the EPICC project utilised every opportunity for participation. This was crucial to showcase the innovative work leading to adoption of the project outputs and resources. Across the duration of the EPICC project, a total of 200 stakeholders participated at the different activities/events. Ultimately, to meet the goal of the EPICC project in promoting excellence in spiritual care education, it was crucial to ensure that all stakeholders had opportunity to participate during the various activities/events.

1.4.1 EPICC Participants

The EPICC project was designed to maximise involvement and engagement of a group of nursing and midwifery educators drawn from higher education institutions across Europe. A balance was achieved between ensuring that as many nursing/midwifery educators as possible from across Europe could participate, whilst providing an intense programme of peer-support, mentorship and coaching. Whilst EPICC Participants collectively formed a distinct group from EPICC Strategic Partners and EPICC Participants+, each Strategic Partner assumed responsibility for

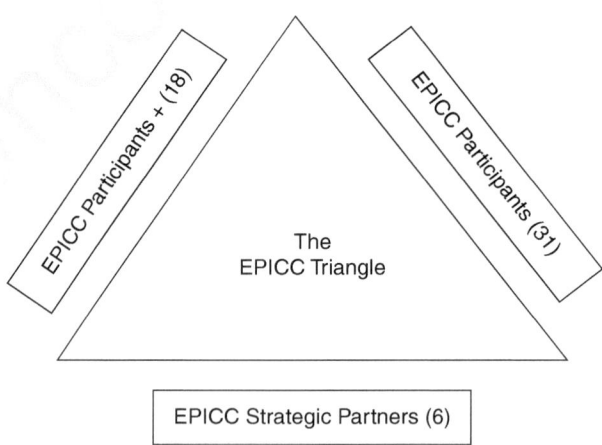

Fig. 1.1 The EPICC triangle

Table 1.2 Participating countries (alphabetical order) (Adapted from McSherry et al. 2020)   t2.1

Belgium	Lithuania	Turkey	t2.2
Croatia	Malta	Ukraine	t2.3
Czech Republic	Norway	United Kingdom (England, Scotland, Wales, Northern	t2.4
Denmark	Poland	Ireland [NI not involved])	t2.5
Germany	Portugal	The Netherlands	t2.6
Greece	Spain	Norway	t2.7
Ireland	Sweden		t2.8

mentoring groups of four to five EPICC Participants throughout the project. This   234
additional level of support fostered trust and respect and helped to prevent attrition   235
of EPICC Participants from the project. This was important for EPICC Participants   236
as they had the most intensive role in the project by testing the development and   237
implementation of various project outputs and resources, such as the EPICC   238
Spiritual Care Education Standard.   239

A wide range of strategies were used to invite EPICC Participants to take part in   240
the project. For example, individuals were identified by the EPICC Strategic Partners   241
through their contacts and extensive networks. An overview of the project was   242
placed on social media, specifically ResearchGate, inviting colleagues to take part,   243
and during the project a closed Facebook group was created to support engagement   244
between the three participating groups. One of the main criteria for participating   245
was attending all the events that formed part of the two cycles of the Action Learning   246
programme. That meant attending both of the two learning/teaching/training activi-   247
ties and two multiplier events. To formally affirm their commitment to the project,   248
all EPICC Participants were required to sign an agreement, indicating that they had   249
sufficient capacity and commitment to participate in the entire project. If they were   250
unable to fulfil this criterion, then alternative EPICC Participants were invited.   251

As mentioned, EPICC Participants represented their higher education institu-   252
tions from across Europe. Most encouraging for the EPICC project was the signifi-   253
cant representation of EPICC Participants, from a total of 21 of the 50 European   254
countries. Table 1.2 presents the countries involved in the EPICC project both   255
directly as participants and indirectly as representatives of key stakeholder groups   256
who were not eligible for funding.   257

1.4.2 EPICC Participants+   258

A key feature of the EPICC project was ensuring that all the key activities, events and   259
outputs were informed by a wide range of cultural, ethnic and religious worldviews.   260
This aim was achieved by the inclusion of a wide range of stakeholders (Participants+).   261
In addition to the examples of stakeholders from various countries within Europe   262
(Table 1.3), the EPICC project comprised Participants+ from five countries outside of   263
Europe (China, Malaysia, New Zealand, Palestine, and Thailand).   264

Table 1.3 Examples of stakeholders in various countries (alphabetical order by country) (Adapted from McSherry et al. 2020)

Country	Stakeholders
China	Staffordshire University
England	NHS England, Public Health England
Malaysia	The National University of Malaysia
Malta	Nursing & Midwifery Board
New Zealand	NorthTec, Whangarei
The Netherlands	Danish Ethical Board, Dutch Higher Education Board
Norway	Norwegian Nursing Association
Palestine	College of Nursing, Islamic University of Gaza
Thailand	Prince of Songkla University
UK	RCN, NHS Chaplaincy
Wales	Welsh Government (Chief Nursing Officer), Health Education Improvement Wales, Social Care Wales, Executive Nurse Directors, Council of Deans Wales, Students

1.5   The Key Activities

The goal of the EPICC project to promote excellence in spiritual care education could only be achieved through a series of key activities that were planned and interspersed across the duration of the project. The key activities are outlined in Table 1.4.

1.6   Methodology

The EPICC project was planned to be both *inclusive* and *participatory*. It was inclusive because it engaged a wide range of groups/stakeholders in a broad range of activities. The participative nature of the project reflected the active involvement and consultation of stakeholders across these activities to achieve the intellectual outputs (Table 1.5). The achievement of various project resources for each intellectual output is indicative of the co-production between the three EPICC groups. From the outset of the project, all the groups remained committed to lead curriculum innovation in how nursing and midwifery education prepares students to address and support spiritual aspects of nursing and midwifery care.

1.6.1   Action Learning

EPICC was conducted using the principles of Action Learning [48]. This is an approach to solving real problems by acting and reflecting upon the results. The learning that resulted from all the different activities and action learning cycles

Table 1.4 Key activities   t4.1

Learning/teaching/training activities (LTTAs) Over 5 days, these project activities comprised large- and small-group work for the 31 EPICC Participants to develop the project outputs	LTTA 1: Viaa Christian University, Zwolle, The Netherlands (October–November 2017). A total of 52 EPICC stakeholders attended LTTA 2 University of Malta, Valletta, Republic of Malta (September 2018). A total of 110 EPICC stakeholders attended	t4.2 t4.3 t4.4 t4.5 t4.6 t4.7
Multiplier events (MEs) Over 2 days, these conference-type events were held at the launch (ME 1) and close (ME 2) of the EPICC project and were organised to share important preparatory information (ME 1) and to share with a wider audience the intellectual outputs that had been generated (ME 2). At ME 2, the EPICC Network was also launched to ensure the legacy of the EPICC project into the future	ME 1: Staffordshire University, United Kingdom (April 2017) with 61 attendees ME 2: University of South Wales, Cardiff, United Kingdom (July 2019) with over 120 attendees	t4.8 t4.9 t4.10 t4.11 t4.12 t4.13 t4.14 t4.15 t4.16 t4.17
Transnational Steering Group Meetings (TNSGs) These were formal meetings to review annual progress, to ensure that the EPICC project remained on target to achieve the intellectual outputs and to ensure the programme was being delivered within the funding envelop	A total of four, TNSGs, involving all EPICC Strategic Partners and a combination of EPICC Participants and Participants+ took place in Zwolle and Ede (The Netherlands) Across the four TNSGs, 51 (30 funded and 21 non-funded) EPICC stakeholders (Strategic Partners, Participants and Participants+) registered attendance	t4.18 t4.19 t4.20 t4.21 t4.22 t4.23 t4.24 t4.25
Monthly and bi-monthly EPICC Strategic Partner and Project Manager Skype meetings Regular Skype mentorship meetings between EPICC Strategic Partners and EPICC Participants in groups of 4–5 Participants	Across the duration of the EPICC project, at least 36 Skype meetings (with agenda) took place EPICC Strategic Partners provided intensive support with their mentor groups, to ensure continued and timely progress	t4.26 t4.27 t4.28 t4.29 t4.30 t4.31

helped improve the problem-solving process and identify potential solutions. For   283
example, EPICC Strategic Partners and EPICC Participants undertook local audits   284
and reviewed and evaluated current educational practice. This comprised mapping   285
of local enablers/inhibitors that impacted on curriculum innovation and change.   286
These activities fostered a culture of mutual support for the exchange of knowledge,   287
expertise and learning. This supportive environment led to the rapid sharing and   288
adoption of good practice within the participating higher education institu-   289
tions (HEIs).   290

The EPICC project was based upon sound educational and pedagogical princi-   291
ples because all the EPICC Strategic Partners and most of the EPICC Participants   292
had extensive experience in nursing and midwifery education, research and prac-   293
tice. Many also had in-depth knowledge, skills and experience in the design and   294
development of nursing and midwifery curricula, along with managing and con-   295
ducting programmes of innovation and change within diverse educational settings.   296

Table 1.5 Intellectual outputs (O)   t5.1

Intellectual output	Description of activity	
O1: Establishing and sustaining the EPICC project	Led by Professor McSherry, and supported by colleagues at Staffordshire University and all the EPICC Strategic Partners, O1 was achieved through raising awareness of the aims and objectives of the EPICC project and strategic partnership internationally and by ensuring the project had a unique brand and identity. The nature and delivery of the project enabled recruitment of a wide range of participants, thus ensuring equality and diversity. Ensuring public, professional regulatory body and stakeholder engagement was crucial, and the effective use of a social media and digital technologies helped to facilitate this. These technologies, along with the development of a bespoke website (www.epicc-network.org) showcased and extended the reach and impact of the EPICC project. The project website primarily serves as a repository for all project resources. Successful planning, implementation and evaluation of all the events and activities were crucial for the success of the project the launch of the EPICC Network	t5.2 t5.3 t5.4 t5.5 t5.6 t5.7 t5.8 t5.9 t5.10 t5.11 t5.12 t5.13 t5.14 t5.15 t5.16 t5.17
O2: Developing a Gold Standard Matrix for Spiritual Care Education and Adoption Toolkit	Led by Professor van Leeuwen, and supported by all the EPICC Strategic Partners, O2 was achieved through developing a Gold Standard Matrix for Spiritual Care Education and Adoption Toolkit. These key project resources focused on (1) enhancement of cultural sensitivity about spirituality and spiritual care; (2) definition of key nursing/midwifery spiritual care competencies; (3) exchange educational practices (learning objectives, learning activities, learning); (4) define key characteristics of an educational matrix for spiritual care; and (5) clarify conditions for implementation and testing of the educational matrix in EPICC Strategic Partners' and EPICC Participants' organisations with the purpose of developing a Matrix and Adoption Toolkit. It was important for Professor van Leeuwen to lead O2 as this enabled him to host and lead LTTA 1. During LTTA 1, a range of activities were undertaken, for example, obtaining EPICC Strategic Partners' and EPICC Participants' feedback from the local mapping and benchmarking audits to identify facilitators and inhibitors. This information was used to co-create the EPICC Gold Standard Matrix for Spiritual Care Education and Adoption Toolkit that was tested as part of the LTTA 2 event in Malta (see below)	t5.18 t5.19 t5.20 t5.21 t5.22 t5.23 t5.24 t5.25 t5.26 t5.27 t5.28 t5.29 t5.30 t5.31 t5.32 t5.33 t5.34 t5.35
O3: Refining and disseminating the Gold Standard Matrix for Spiritual Care Education and Adoption Toolkit	Led by Dr. Attard, and supported by all the EPICC Strategic Partners, O3 was achieved through capturing the experiences and sharing best practice between EPICC groups about the implementation of the EPICC Matrix and Adoption Toolkit. An important part of this process was to identify the facilitators and inhibitors reported by EPICC Participants who had tested the EPICC Matrix and strategies for the Adoption Toolkit. Having participants from 21 European countries was a significant strength when developing and refining these resources. This enabled resources to be interpreted in their respective cultures. It was important for Dr. Attard to lead O3 as this enabled her to host and lead LTTA 2. During LTTA 2, EPICC Participants were supported to prepare for the local implementation and adoption of the refined EPICC Matrix and Adoption Toolkit. LTTA 2 proved to be a source of inspiration for Participants, with opportunities to report on the implementation and integration of the EPICC Spiritual Care Education Standard into existing or new nursing/midwifery curricula, along with preliminary results of success and challenges	t5.36 t5.37 t5.38 t5.39 t5.40 t5.41 t5.42 t5.43 t5.44 t5.45 t5.46 t5.47 t5.48 t5.49 t5.50 t5.51

1.6.2   Intellectual Outputs   297

All EPICC Strategic Partners utilised their extensive expertise in designing and   298
delivering programmes of education and spiritual care education. This knowledge   299
and experience were fundamental to leading and achieving the different intellectual 300
outputs (Table 1.5). The EPICC Strategic Partners' expertise was maximised by   301
ensuring developmental work towards each of the intellectual outputs was mapped   302
against previous research and educational practice. Therefore, all the associated   303
activities assigned to the different intellectual outputs complemented their expertise 304
and played to their individual strengths.   305

Activities were purposefully designed to build upon each other, incrementally   306
creating a culture where EPICC Strategic Partners could facilitate learning and sup- 307
port for all the EPICC Participants. This learning was informed by the voice and   308
experiences of the EPICC Participants+ who reviewed and critiqued the develop-   309
ments and outputs from the EPICC project, ensuring they were fit for purpose and   310
practice.   311

The opportunity for all the EPICC participant groups to network with each other   312
and share knowledge and experiences was of crucial importance in establishing a   313
sense of community whilst accommodating each other's different national, cultural   314
and professional backgrounds. Throughout every stage of the EPICC project, all   315
groups demonstrated a willingness and desire to learn from each through their   316
shared vision to achieve all the intellectual outputs. Project events and activities 317
allowed EPICC Strategic Partners to monitor progress and adjust direction if neces- 318
sary. The developmental nature of the events and activities supported the achieve-   319
ment of the three intellectual outputs, which were shared at the final project event 320
(multiplier event 2) along with the launch of the EPICC Network.   321

1.7   Outputs and Achievements   322

The synergistic way of working outlined above helped to reduce costs and promoted   323
greater cooperation, creating clear lines of governance and reinforcing accountabil- 324
ity. The interactive and cyclic nature of the events meant that all intellectual outputs 325
were co-created throughout the duration of the EPICC project. In addition, creative 326
approaches were used to evaluate the usefulness and potential impact of the outputs. 327
These included the use of Post-it® notes to capture words that described delegates' 328
thoughts and feelings at the end of activities/events. Electronic questionnaires (via 329
email) were used to assess respondents' satisfaction. At the end of the project, a   330
60-item, Likert scale evaluation questionnaire was sent to all EPICC Participants,   331
which sought to capture their involvement with the project by addressing: (1) the   332
content of the EPICC Spiritual Care Education Standard; (2) the usefulness of the   333
EPICC Gold Standard Matrix (and narrative) and (3) their involvement in achieving   334
the project aims and outcomes.   335

At the end of the evaluation questionnaire was one open question that enabled respondents to share any final reflections of their involvement with the project. Overall, this evaluation provided excellent quantitative and qualitative data regarding the governance and quality of the project and has been used to inform the final report submitted to the UK National Agency.

Collectively these strategies ensured the co-creation of the following key outputs:

1. EPICC Gold Standard Matrix for Spiritual Care Education.
2. EPICC Gold Standard Matrix for Spiritual Care Education Narrative to the Matrix.
3. EPICC Spiritual Care Education Standard.
4. EPICC Adoption Toolkit.

A brief overview of the outputs is provided below along with links to access and download these resources from the EPICC website (www.epicc-network. org) for free.

1.7.1 *EPICC Gold Standard Matrix for Spiritual Care Education and Narrative to the Matrix*

The EPICC Matrix (link https://blogs.staffs.ac.uk/epicc/files/2019/06/EPICC-Gold-Standard-Matrix-for-Spiritual-Care-Education.pdf) and its accompanying narrative (https://blogs.staffs.ac.uk/epicc/files/2019/06/EPICC-Gold-Standard-Matrix-Narrative.pdf) outline the cultural, social and political environment in which spiritual care competency develops. They detail the factors that need to be considered such as a student's values, attitudes and behaviours concerning spirituality and spiritual care. It also outlines the institutional and organisational factors that impact students' development in providing spiritual care. An in-depth understanding of these is necessary if one is to foster environments and cultures where students can acquire the requisite knowledge, skills and attitudes to feel confident and competent in the delivery of spiritual care.

1.7.2 *EPICC Spiritual Care Education Standard*

The 'EPICC Standard' (https://blogs.staffs.ac.uk/epicc/files/2019/06/EPICC-Spiritual-Care-Education-Standard.pdf) details a table of four key spiritual care competencies expected from undergraduate/preregistration nursing and midwifery students. The table of competencies is preceded by a preamble containing important information, such as how spirituality is defined and what is meant by spiritual care. In addition, some explanatory notes are provided in relation to the cultural context and terminology used throughout the Standard.

For every competence, the learning outcomes are described in aspects of knowledge (*cognitive*), skills (*functional*) and attitudes (*behavioural*). The underpinning
philosophy is that these competencies are practiced within a compassionate relationship and founded in a person-centred and reflective attitude of openness, presence and trust, that is fundamental for nursing and midwifery.

- *For an overview of the process and steps involved in the development of the four
  competences, please see Suggested Reading. (McSherry et al. 2020, 62)*

Each of the four competencies is addressed in-depth in subsequent chapters of
the book. Chapter 5 addresses Competence 1: Intrapersonal Spirituality, where the
student *is aware of the importance of spirituality on health and well-being*. Chapter
6 addresses Competence 2: Interpersonal Spirituality, where the student *engages
with persons' spirituality, acknowledging their unique spiritual and cultural worldviews, beliefs and practices*. Chapters 7 and 8 deal with the delivery of spiritual.
Chapter 7 addresses Competence 3: Assessment and Planning, where the student
*assesses spiritual needs and resources using appropriate formal or informal
approaches, and plans spiritual care, maintaining confidentiality and obtaining
informed consent*. Chapter 8 addresses Competence 4: Intervention and Evaluation,
where the student *responds to spiritual needs and resources within a caring, compassionate relationship*.

1.7.3 EPICC Adoption Toolkit

Development of the EPICC Toolkit (http://blogs.staffs.ac.uk/epicc/resources/epicc-
adoption-toolkit/) involved several phases. During multiplier event 1, participants
were asked to share and present examples of the educational resources and strategies that they used in the teaching of spiritual care. This was further developed at the
first learning/teaching/training activity, where EPICC Participants were invited to
produce posters of one teaching/learning activity. Posters had to contain adequate
details to enable the utility and replicability of the activity by other nursing/mid-
wifery educators. Such details included having a title, teaching strategy, learning
objectives, detailed description of activity, educator's role, resources, assessment
details, and references.

Throughout the duration of the EPICC project, all three groups (not just Participants)
contributed to the Toolkit. All educational strategies used in the Toolkit were reviewed
and aligned with one or more of the four competencies as per the EPICC Standard. The
aim of this approach was to make it relatively straightforward for educators when
selecting a range of strategies to support their teaching of various competencies. One
EPICC Participant+ also provided a generic educational strategy in the teaching of
spiritual care, that has not been categorised under the four competencies in the EPICC
Standard (https://blogs.staffs.ac.uk/epicc/files/2019/06/25-JP.pdf).

409   • *Crucially, the EPICC Adoption Toolkit is a live resource, meaning individuals*
410   *can constantly add new and innovative activities, so that the range and reper-*
411   *toire of the toolkit can be expanded.*

1.8   Overview of the Book

413   Chapter 2 explores the different elements of spirituality and spiritual care such as
414   what is meant by the terms *existential, religious, life events* and *suffering*. It pro-
415   vides an overview of the many views of what it means to be a human being. Finally,
416   it discusses what is understood by spirituality and spiritual care both within a
417   European and international context. Chapter 3 delves into the educational context
418   and evidence. By drawing upon international evidence, this chapter explores the
419   need for nurses/midwives to be competent in spiritual care to meet expectations of
420   nursing/midwifery regulatory bodies, professional educational guidelines, and to
421   respond to the patient/client/carer voice. Chapter 4 is titled 'Self-Care', since it was
422   felt imperative that in order to manage and remain sensitive to patients' needs and
423   sufferings, then those providing care must be in a position to care for themselves
424   physically, psychologically, socially, and spiritually. Chapters 5–8 deal with the
425   four individual competencies for spiritual care respectively as previously detailed in
426   Sect. 1.7.2. Finally, Chapter 9 presents a summary of the impact of the EPICC proj-
427   ect and the ongoing developments for the EPICC Network.

1.9   Summary

429   The EPICC project has informed the delivery of nursing/midwifery education inter-
430   nationally and will continue to enhance the quality and skill set of student nurses/
431   midwives in participating institutions as the intellectual outputs and resources
432   become embedded in programmes. This will ensure that students have the profes-
433   sional values, attitudes and behaviours to provide high-quality, compassionate and
434   safe nursing/midwifery care. In the long term, EPICC will ensure a consistent
435   approach to teaching and learning about spiritual aspects of care. Part of the EPICC
436   journey has been documented in this chapter and events and activities recorded on
437   the EPICC website providing an historical record of the work undertaken and the
438   significant achievements.
439   The focus of the EPICC project on ensuring that undergraduate nurse and mid-
440   wives possess the correct knowledge, skill and attitudes will ensure all nursing and
441   midwifery care is more holistic, humanistic, compassionate and person-centred.
442   This refocusing of attitudes, values and behaviours will hopefully prevent reoccur-
443   rence of situations where there have been concerns about poor standards of care,
444   where there has been a lack of compassion and respect for patients' dignity, result-
445   ing in unnecessary patient suffering and deaths.

The primary legacy of the EPICC project is establishing of the EPICC 446
Network. This will continue to direct, shape and influence nursing/midwifery 447
education, research and practice globally. The main beneficiaries of EPICC who 448
were not directly involved but will benefit are patients receiving nursing and 449
midwifery care in institutions associated and affiliated to the project. The four 450
key outputs from EPICC have already started to have some direct impact by 451
raising awareness of the importance of spiritual aspects of nursing and mid- 452
wifery practice through curriculum innovation. The improvements in nursing 453
and midwifery education being advocated and promoted as a part of EPICC 454
project will ensure that nursing, midwifery and healthcare in general becomes 455
more holistic and person-centred, putting the patient and public back at the cen- 456
tre of all care delivery. 457

References 458

1. European Association for Palliative Care. Spiritual care. 2011. www.eapcnet.eu/eapc-groups/ 459
reference/spiritual-care. Accessed 18 Nov 2019. 460
2. Puchalski CM, Vitillo R, Hull SK, Reller N. Improving the spiritual dimension of whole per- 461
son care: reaching national and international consensus. J Palliat Med. 2014;17(6):642–56. 462
https://doi.org/10.1089/jpm.2014.9427. 463
3. Weathers E, McCarthy G, Coffey A. Concept analysis of spirituality: an evolutionary approach. 464
Nurs Forum. 2016;51(2):79–96. https://doi.org/10.1111/nuf.12128. 465
4. Murgia C, Notarnicola I, Rocco G, Stievano A. Spirituality in nursing: a concept analysis. Nurs 466
Ethics. 2020. https://doi.org/10.1177/0969733020909534. 467
5. European Commission. Europe 2020: a strategy for smart, sustainable and inclusive growth. 468
2010. https://ec.europa.eu/eu2020/pdf/COMPLET%20EN%20BARROSO%20%20%20 469
007%20-%20Europe%202020%20-%20EN%20version.pdf. Accessed 18 Nov 2019. 470
6. National Health Service (NHS) England. NHS Chaplaincy guidelines 2015: promoting excel- 471
lence in pastoral, spiritual & religious care. Leeds: NHS England; 2015. https://www.eng- 472
land.nhs.uk/wp-content/uploads/2015/03/nhs-chaplaincyguidelines-2015.pdf. Accessed 18 473
Nov 2019. 474
7. Norwegian Health Library. Åndelige og eksistensielle behov hos pasienter og pårørende 475
(Spiritual and existential needs of patients and relatives). 2019. https://www.helsebiblioteket. 476
no/fagprosedyrer/ferdige/andelige-og-eksistensielle-behov-hospasienter-og-parorende. 477
Accessed 18 Nov 2019. 478
8. Norwegian Helsedirektoratet. Nasjonalt handlingsprogram for palliasjon I kreftomsorgen: 479
Nasjonal faglig retningslinje IS-2800 (National Action Program for Palliation in Cancer 480
Care: National Academic Guideline: IS-2800). 2015. https://www.helsedirektoratet.no/ret- 481
ningslinjer/palliasjon-i-kreftomsorgen-handlingsprogram/Palliasjon%20i%20kreftomsor- 482
gen%20-%20Nasjonalt%20handlingsprogram%20med%20retningslinjer.pdf/_/attachment/ 483
inline/95636e37-ce73-4f2f-a61d-ee3f9e1ccada:fd30165370557eebcb60adcdb8473e4b78 484
6776b4/Palliasjon%20i%20kreftomsorgen%20-%20Nasjonalt%20handlingsprogram%20 485
med%20retningslinjer.pdf. Accessed 18 Nov 2019. 486
9. The Scottish Government. Spiritual care & chaplaincy. 2009. https://www.nes.scot.nhs.uk/ 487
media/3688/Spiritual-Car-%20and-Chaplaincy.pdf. Accessed 18 Nov 2019. 488
10. Welsh Government. Health and care standards. 2015. http://www.wales.nhs.uk/sitesplus/ 489
documents/1064/24729%5FHealth%20Standards%20Framework%5F2015%5FE1.pdf. 490
Accessed 18 Nov 2019. 491

11. Balboni TA, Fitchett G, Handzo GF, Johnson KS, Koenig HG, Pargament KI, Puchalski CM, Sinclair S, Taylor EJ, Steinhauser KE. State of the science of spirituality and palliative care research part ii: screening, assessment, and interventions. J Pain Symptom Manage. 2017;54(3):441–53. https://doi.org/10.1016/j.jpainsymman.2017.07.029.

12. Koenig H, King DE, Carson VB. Handbook of religion and health. 2nd ed. New York: Oxford University Press; 2012.

13. Steinhauser KE, Fitchett G, Handzo GF, Johnson KS, Koenig HG, Pargament KI, Puchalski CM, Sinclair S, Taylor EJ, Balboni TA. State of the science of spirituality and palliative care research part i: definitions, measurement, and outcomes. J Pain Symptom Manage. 2017;54(3):428–40. https://doi.org/10.1016/j.jpainsymman.2017.07.028.

14. Giske T, Cone PH. Discerning the healing pat: how nurses assist patients spiritually in diverse health care settings. J Clin Nurs. 2015;24(19–20):2926–35. https://doi.org/10.1111/jocn.12907.

15. Ross L. Spiritual care in nursing: an overview of the research to date. J Clin Nurs. 2006;15(7):852–62. https://doi.org/10.1111/j.1365-2702.2006.01617.x.

16. Ross L, Austin J. Spiritual needs and spiritual support preferences of people with end-stage heart failure and their carers: implications for nurse managers. J Nurs Manag. 2015;23(1):87–95. https://doi.org/10.1111/jonm.12087.

17. Selman LE, Brighton LJ, Sinclair S, Karvinen I, Egan R, Speck P, Powell RA, et al. Patients' and caregivers' needs, experiences, preferences and research priorities in spiritual care: a focus group study across nine countries. Palliat Med. 2018;32(1):216–30. https://doi.org/10.1177/0269216317734954.

18. Department of Health. End of life care strategy: promoting high quality care for all adults at the end of life. 2008. https://www.gov.uk/government/publications/end-of-life-care-strategy-promoting-high-quality-care-for-adults-at-the-end-of-their-life.

19. Marie Curie Cancer Care (MCCC). Spiritual and religious care competencies for specialist palliative care. London: Marie Curie Cancer Care; 2003. http://www.ahpcc.org.uk/pdf/spirit-comp.pdf?LMCL=PSkgiT. Accessed 18 Nov 2019.

20. NHS Education Scotland (NES). Spiritual care matters: an introductory resource for all NHS Scotland Staff. Edinburgh: NHS Education for Scotland; 2009. https://www.nes.scot.nhs.uk/media/3723/spiritualcaremattersfinal.pdf. Accessed 18 Nov 2019.

21. Royal College of Physicians (RCP). End of Life Care Audit—dying in hospital: National Report for England 2016. 2016. https://www.rcplondon.ac.uk/projects/outputs/end-life-care-audit-dying-hospital-national-report-england-2016. Accessed 18 Nov 2019.

22. Dementia Services Development Centre. Trusted to care: 2015 review. 2015. http://www.wales.nhs.uk/sitesplus/documents/863/TrustedtoCareReview2015final%20%281%29.pdf. Accessed 18 Nov 2019.

23. Department of Health. Winterbourne View Hospital: Department of Health Review and Response. 2012. https://www.gov.uk/government/publications/winterbourne-view-hospital-department-of-health-review-and-response. Accessed 18 Nov 2019.

24. The Mid Staffordshire NHS Foundation Trust Public Inquiry. Report of the Mid Staffordshire NHS Foundation Trust Public Inquiry. 2013. https://webarchive.nationalarchives.gov.uk/20150407084003/http://www.midstaffspublicinquiry.com/. Accessed 18 Nov 2019.

25. The Patients Association. Patients…not numbers, people…not statistics. 2009. https://www.patientlibrary.net/tempgen/5361.pdf. Accessed 18 Nov 2019.

26. The Patients Association. Listen to patients, speak up for change. 2010. https://www.annerobsontrust.org.uk/wp-content/uploads/2018/06/Listen-to-patients-Speak-up-for-change.pdf. Accessed 18 Nov 2019.

27. The Patients Association. We've been listening, have you been learning? 2011. https://www.west-info.eu/grandpas-got-into-the-wrong-elderly-care-patientshospital-health-care-united-kingdom/weve-been-listening-have-you-been-learning/. Accessed 18 Nov 2019.

28. Ali G, Snowden M, Wattis J, Rogers M. Spirituality in nursing education: knowledge and practice gaps. Int J Multidiscip Comparat Stud. 2018;5(1–3):27–49.

29. Fenton E, Mitchell T. Growing old with dignity: a concept analysis. Nurs Pract. 2002;14(4):19–21. https://doi.org/10.7748/nop2002.06.14.4.19.c2212.

30. Lewinson LP. The impact of pre-registration nurses' spirituality education on clinical practice: a grounded theory investigation. PhD dissertation. Staffordshire University, 2016.
31. International Confederation of Midwives. International code of ethics for midwives. 2008. https://www.internationalmidwives.org/assets/files/general-files/2019/01/cd2008_001-eng-code-of-ethics-for-midwives.pdf. Accessed 18 Nov 2019.
32. International Council of Nurses. The ICN code of ethics for nurses. 2012. https://www.icn.ch/sites/default/files/inline-files/2012_ICN_Codeofethicsfornurses_%20eng.pdf.
33. Ministry of Education and Research (Norway). Forskrift om Felles rammeplan for helse og sosialutdanningene (Regulations on a common framework plan for health and social science education). 2017. https://lovdata.no/dokument/SF/forskrift/2017-09-06-1353. Accessed 18 Nov 2019.
34. Nursing and Midwifery Council (NMC). Future nurse: standards of proficiency for registered nurses. 2018. https://www.nmc.org.uk/standards/standards-for-nurses/standards-of-proficiency-for-registered-nurses/. Accessed 18 Nov 2019.
35. Royal College of Nursing (RCN). Spirituality survey 2010. 2011. https://www.rcn.org.uk/professional-development/publications/pub-003861. Accessed 18 Nov 2019.
36. Lewinson L, McSherry W, Kevern P. Spirituality in pre-registration nurse education and practice: a review of the literature. Nurse Educ Today. 2015;35:806–14.
37. Lewinson LP, McSherry W, Kevern P. "Enablement"—spirituality engagement in pre-registration nurse education and practice: a grounded theory investigation. Religions. 2018;9(11):1–14. https://doi.org/10.3390/rel9110356.
38. Ross LA. Spiritual aspects of nursing. J Adv Nurs. 1994;19(3):439–47. https://doi.org/10.1111/j.1365-2648.1994.tb01105.x.
39. Egan R, Llewellyn R, Cox B, MacLeod R, McSherry W, Austin P. New Zealand Nurses' perceptions of spirituality and spiritual care: qualitative findings from a national survey. Religions. 2017;8(5):79. https://doi.org/10.3390/rel8050079.
40. McSherry W, Gretton M, Draper P, Watson R. The ethical basis of teaching spirituality and spiritual care: A survey of student nurses perceptions. Nurse Education Today. 2008;28(8):1002–1008.
41. Ross L, Giske T, van Leeuwen R, Baldacchino D, McSherry W, Narayanasamy A, Jarvis P, Schep-Akkerman A. Factors contributing to student nurses'/midwives' perceived competency in spiritual care. Nurse Educ Today. 2016;36:445–51. https://doi.org/10.1016/j.nedt.2015.10.005.
42. Ross L, van Leeuwen R, Baldacchino D, Giske T, McSherry W, Narayanasamy A, Downes C, Jarvis P, Schep-Akkerman A. Student nurses perceptions of spirituality and competence in delivering spiritual care: a European Pilot Study. Nurse Educ Today. 2014;34(5):697–702. https://doi.org/10.1016/j.nedt.2013.09.014.
43. McSherry W, Draper P, Kendrick D. Construct validity of a rating scale designed to assess spirituality and spiritual care. Int J Nurs Stud. 2002;39(7):723–34. https://doi.org/10.1016/S0020-7489(02)00014-7.
44. Van Leeuwen R, Tiesinga LJ, Middel B, Post D, Jochemsen H. The validity and reliability of an instrument to assess nursing competencies in spiritual care. J Clin Nurs. 2009;18(20):2857–69. https://doi.org/10.1111/j.1365-2702.2008.02594.x.
45. Ross L, McSherry W, Giske T, van Leeuwen R, Schep-Akkerman A, Koslander T, Hall J, Steenfeldt VØ, Jarvis P. Nursing and midwifery students' perceptions of spirituality, spiritual care, and spiritual care competency: a prospective, longitudinal, correlational European study. Nurse Educ Today. 2018;67:64–71. https://doi.org/10.1016/j.nedt.2018.05.002.
46. Attard J, Ross L, Weeks KW. Design and development of a spiritual care competency framework for pre-registration nurses and midwives: a modified Delphi Study. Nurse Educ Pract. 2019;39:96–104. https://doi.org/10.1016/j.nepr.2019.08.003.
47. Erasmus+: Glossary | Erasmus+. n.d. https://www.erasmusplus.org.uk/glossary. Accessed 19 Jun 2020.
48. Revans RW. ABC's of action learning. Burlington: Gower Publishing; 2011.

Suggested Reading

For an overview of the project please visit the EPICC Project website at http://www.epicc-network.org

The following article provides a useful summary of the EPICC Project and complements this chapter:

McSherry W, Ross L, Attard J, van Leeuwen R, Giske T, Kleiven T, Boughey A, the EPICC Network. Preparing undergraduate nurses and midwives for spiritual care: some developments in European education over the last decade. J Study Spirituality. 2020;10(1):55–71. https://doi.org/10.1080/20440243.2020.1726053.

Chapter 2
What Do We Mean by 'Spirituality' and 'Spiritual Care'?

Tormod Kleiven, Bart Cusveller, Marianne Rodriguez Nygaard,
Štefica Mikšić, Adam Boughey, and Wilfred McSherry

> **Learning Objectives**
> This chapter will enable you to:
>
> 1. Identify the different elements of spirituality and reflect on some phenom-
>   enological (lived experience) aspects of spirituality.

T. Kleiven (✉)
VID Specialized University, Oslo, Norway
e-mail: tormod.kleiven@vid.no

B. Cusveller
Academy of Health Care, and Spiritual Care in Nursing Research Institute (lectorate),
Viaa Christian University of Applied Sciences, Zwolle, The Netherlands
e-mail: b.cusveller@viaa.nl

M. R. Nygaard
Diakonia and Leadership Studies, VID Specialized University,
Oslo, Norway
e-mail: marianne.rodriguez.nygaard@vid.no

Š. Mikšić
Department of Nursing and Palliative Medicine, Faculty of Dental Medicine
and Health Osijek, Josip Juraj Strossmayer of Osijek, Osijek, Croatia
e-mail: smiksic@fdmz.hr

A. Boughey
Department of Nursing, School of Health and Social Care, Staffordshire University,
Stoke-on-Trent, Staffordshire, England, UK
e-mail: adam.boughey@staffs.ac.uk

W. McSherry
Department of Nursing, School of Health and Social Care, University Hospitals of North
Midlands NHS Trust, Staffordshire University, Stoke-on-Trent, Staffordshire, England, UK

VID University College, Bergen/Oslo, Norway
e-mail: w.mcsherry@staffs.ac.uk

© Springer Nature Switzerland AG 2021
W. McSherry et al. (eds.), *Enhancing Nurses' and Midwives' Competence in
Providing Spiritual Care*, https://doi.org/10.1007/978-3-030-65888-5_2

2. Understand the concept of spiritual care and how an awareness or an omission of this might affect the quality of nursing/midwifery care.
3. Reflect on and discuss key aspects of spirituality and spiritual care in the European and international contexts.

2.1 Introduction

As this book focuses on the enhancement of nurses' and midwives' competence in providing spiritual care through innovative education and compassionate care, it is important to orientate to the notions of *spirituality* and *spiritual care*. Understanding the content and application of these terms in respect of their relevance to nursing and midwifery is crucial to actively engage with the following chapters.

Over the past 40 years, the study of spirituality and spiritual care has become significant areas of scientific research not just within the classical disciplines such as theology and philosophy but increasingly within healthcare practice. The aim of this chapter is to provide some helpful descriptions and reflections regarding the terms. It will also offer some overarching reflections and theoretical references in how to understand spirituality and spiritual care in nursing and midwifery. Two practice examples will be provided: (1) to illustrate the positive effect of providing spiritual care; and (2) when spiritual care is lacking and the consequent negative impact on a patient. This introductory discussion will be explored more fully in the following chapters.

The chapter starts with a discussion of spirituality as a term and as a phenomenon against the background of the EPICC project (www.epicc-project.eu). This is a precursor to further discussion and elaboration that focuses on the phenomenological (lived experience) aspects of how we perceive what it is to be a human being. Of course, as this book is focused on enhancing nurses' and midwives' competence in providing spiritual care, just focusing on the aforementioned theoretical discussion would not be sufficient. Therefore, this chapter also exemplifies and describes what spiritual care is about and how it can be provided. Throughout the chapter, readers might have considered the importance of understanding spirituality and spiritual care within different national, social and cultural contexts. We have acknowledged the significance of this and offer some final discussion in respect of spiritual care as it pertains to the European and international contexts.

A cautionary note: while every effort has been made to capture the complexity of spirituality in the European context, there may be published or unpublished work that the authors are not aware of that offer important insights into the specifics of spiritual care delivery for certain European countries/regions.

Throughout the chapter, we encourage you to make some notes of personal reflections on spirituality and spiritual care as relevant to your country, culture and healthcare practice (if applicable). We aim that the information provided in this chapter will help to orientate readers to the concepts of spirituality and spiritual care

as the foundation for understanding information in the following chapters. However,   42
it is likely that your own notes and reflections will also serve as important learning   43
materials.   44

2.2   Spirituality: As a Term and Phenomenon   45

This section concludes with a working definition of spirituality that was adopted by   46
the EPICC project and published in the preamble to the EPICC Spiritual Care   47
Education Standard.[1] This is the consensus-based definition adapted from the   48
European Association for Palliative Care that was first developed by Puchalski   49
et al. [1].   50

2.2.1   Many Definitions   51

Before stating this working definition of spirituality, it is worth outlining some   52
definitions published in the nursing and midwifery literature (Table 2.1). These   53
definitions raise two important questions that need to be answered throughout this   54
section.   55
The definitions above raise a number of questions, the first question being: 56

- What is the *phenomenon* that these definitions try to point to?   57
- Or simply: what are they about? Like Hay [7] in the title of his book *Something*   58
  There. So, what is this 'something there' and can it be defined and explained (can   59
  we 'put our finger on it')? It is often suggested spirituality 'does' this or that, or   60
  'has' such and such. Nevertheless, what is 'it' and what does it 'do'?   61

The second question is: 62

- What definition will be used in this book? We will come back to this after answer-   63
  ing the first question.   64

Activity 1
Please can you read through the definitions presented in Table 2.1. *Write down any common aspects, such as words that appear in all the definitions, or if you have considered any patterns in human reality that gives the term 'spirituality' some grounding.*

---

[1] Available: https://blogs.staffs.ac.uk/epicc/files/2020/08/EPICC-Spiritual-Care-Education-Standard.pdf

Table 2.1 Definitions of spirituality

Author(s), (year), page	Definition
Nash and Yuen [2]	Spirituality can be defined as a sensitivity or attachment to religious or other values that helps a person gain insight, self-knowledge, and a heightened understanding of life
Puchalski and Ferrell [3], p. 25	Spirituality is the aspect of humanity that refers to the way individuals seek and express meaning and purpose and the way they experience their connectedness to the moment, to self, to others, to nature, and to the significant or sacred
Koenig et al. [4], p. 46	Spirituality is distinguished from other things—Humanism, values, morals, and mental health—By its connection to that which is sacred, the *transcendent*. The transcendent is that which is outside of the self, and yet also within the self—And in Western traditions is called god, Allah, HaShem or a higher power, and in eastern traditions may be called Brahman, manifestations of Brahman, Buddha, Dao, or ultimate truth/reality. Spirituality is intimately connected to the supernatural, the mystical, and to organized religion, although it also extends beyond organized religion (and begins before it). Spirituality includes both a search for the transcendent and the discovery of the transcendent, and so involves traveling along the path that leads from nonconsideration to questioning to ether staunch non-belief or belief, and if belief, then ultimately to a devotion, and finally surrender
Canfield et al. [5], p. 206	[spirituality in health care is] that part of person that gives meaning and purpose to the person's life. Belief in a higher power that may inspire hope, seek resolution, and transcend physical and conscious constraints
Crowther and Hall [6], p. 175	Spirituality and spiritual care is 'being with another' as midwives walk with mothers and is embedded in all that midwives do

Your review of the definitions may have revealed various patterns across the different definitions, such as how people find meaning and purpose in life, and the concept of transcendence which is having an awareness of being part of something greater than yourself. For some people, this may be found in their religious beliefs and practice. It is about connections and relationships with other people and with the environment. It also concerns what we believe in and for some people this may be God or a deity. While for others, it may be a sense of being part of creation or the natural environment. Some of these points will be explored in the following section.

Before proceeding to the next section, we would like to explore with you in a little more detail the differences and similarities between two words: 'existential' and 'spiritual' that are used in health care that seem to be describing or pointing to the same thing. In Table 2.2, we have presented two definitions in respect of these terms.

Activity 2

Reflect upon the words 'spiritual' and 'existential'. Are there any differences in how these two words are used to describe the notion of spirituality?

Table 2.2 Spiritual or existential   t2.1

Term	Definition	Author(s), (year), page	
Spiritual	Spirituality is the aspect of humanity that refers to the way individuals seek and express meaning and purpose and the way they experience their connectedness to the moment, to self, to others, to nature, and to the significant or sacred	Puchalski and Ferrell [3], p. 25	t2.2 t2.3 t2.4 t2.5 t2.6 t2.7
Existential	The existential dimension is focused on the individual's understanding of existentiality and the way meaning is created. This dimension includes the worldview conception, life approach, decision-making structure, way of relating, and way of understanding. It also includes the activities of expressions of symbolic significance, such as rituals and other ways of making meaning	DeMarinis [8], pp. 44–45	t2.8 t2.9 t2.10 t2.11 t2.12 t2.13 t2.14

The reason why we are introducing you to these concepts is because in some   78
countries the word existential seems to be used more commonly than the word spiri-   79
tual. This maybe because of issues associated with language and translation of the   80
word spiritual. Table 2.2 offers a definition of spiritual and existential. Please read   81
through these definitions, comparing the words and phrases used to define them.   82
You may want to highlight any differences or similarities. You may also ask yourself   83
whether one (or both) definition(s) are best suited for nursing and midwifery   84
practice.   85

2.2.2   *What the Definitions Are About?*   86

As we see it, understanding spirituality involves a number of steps. Step 1 refers to   87
spirituality an experience, namely the awareness we have of our 'human condition'.   88
By this 'human condition' we mean the 'inevitable givens' or 'basic conditions' of   89
life, like the fact of being born, being mortal, being vulnerable, being male or   90
female, being a parent and child, being embodied, being in history and in society,   91
being part of a larger whole (cosmic, sacred) and so on. Most of the time, we just   92
take these structural facts of human existence for granted. In any sort of circum-   93
stance, for instance in the case of suffering, we may be conscious of this existential   94
experience. This we call spirituality.   95

The definitions of spirituality also highlight that, in step 2, individuals are   96
engaged in what we may also call or refer to as *practices* of relating to the funda-   97
mentals of human life. For example, seeking or expressing it through rituals, intro-   98
spection and/or a devout lifestyle. Therefore, a person's *experience* and the *practice*   99
of spirituality may then go together.   100

This experience will usually accord with an *evaluation* of one's human condi-   101
tion. This means that we do not just experience our existence as it comes, but also   102
experience it (or not) as consistent, valuable, meaningful and so on. That is why we   103
often talk about spirituality in terms of 'existential meaning' or more precisely, the   104

experience of existential meaning. Whether or not we experience, for instance, suffering as meaningful depends on one's context. Perhaps meaning is most often experienced in connection to something outside oneself, like significant others, nature, work, art and so on. This may also include connection to 'a larger whole', 'wholly other(s)' and/or God. Baumiller [9] suggested that giving birth may bring women who are identified as religious closer to the Higher Being they believe in. During birth, the Higher Being is viewed as able to influence birth, along with a transformative experience where birth becomes more meaningful and religious ritual may be used as a coping mechanism [10].

Let us single out for attention here that these first two points—spirituality as experience and spirituality as experience of existential meaning—will often relate to one's health and hence to the context of impaired health, and provision of health care. This means that spirituality is not a nice extra nor a bothersome obligation but, rather, that its presence in health, well-being and provision of compassionate health care is inevitable. It is therefore not only useful to attend to spirituality in the caring and helping processes of nursing and midwifery, but also that the patient is deserving of this attention to their spirituality and spiritual well-being as a fundamental aspect of their humanity.

In step 3, it is of clinical relevance to note that these experiences (and practices) of spirituality are most often expressed in (parts of) religious language. Patients talk of hope, trust, connectedness, thankfulness and so on, and it matters a good deal for many patients that these concepts have their origin and can be made sense of in the context of their religious affiliations. So, even if people do not experience 'meaning' (be it spiritual and/or existential) through organised religions (for example, church membership or church attendance), it is important for nurses/midwives to realise that a specific patient's spiritual experiences and practices may still be informed in some way by religion in one's personal and cultural communities and traditions. Therefore, nurses'/midwives' knowledge of world religions, for instance, may help them to provide effective, skilled and compassionate spiritual care.

2.2.3   A Working Definition

After establishing that spirituality is an experience of 'the facts of life', it may be no surprise that there are many definitions. Definitions of spirituality can focus on different aspects or different groups' ideas of spirituality. For the purpose of this book, we do *not* have to decide what 'the best' definition of spirituality is (if indeed there is one). Instead, nursing and midwifery students will appreciate that the EPICC project, and its legacy as the EPICC network, offers a pragmatic choice for a working definition of spirituality.

Pragmatically, what might we consider to be, not necessarily the *best*, but a *good* (practical) working definition? The definition should preferably be in-line with the view of spirituality explained above and should be relevant to application in the context of health care; based on research, expertise and consensus among recognised experts. Within the context of health care, comprehensive and practical

definitions of spirituality have often been focused within palliative care. Therefore,   147
the EPICC project (and its subsequent EPICC network) has adopted a definition   148
developed by the European Association for Palliative Care [11]:   149

> *Spirituality is the dynamic dimension of human life that relates to the way persons (indi-*   150
> *vidual and community) experience, express and/or seek meaning, purpose and transcen-*   151
> *dence, and the way they connect to the moment, to self, to others, to nature, to the significant*   152
> *and/or the sacred.*   153

Considering the various definitions of spirituality mentioned previously in Sect.   154
2.2.1, the above EAPC definition helps to address the first question (the *phenome-*   155
non of spirituality) and also the second question (adopting a definition for the pur-   156
pose of the EPICC project and network). To adopt this definition, the EPICC project   157
and network has itself reached consensus on the following considerations, which   158
feature in the preamble of the EPICC Spiritual Care Education Standard: 159

> *The spiritual field is multidimensional:*   160
> *   1. Existential challenges (e.g., questions concerning identity, meaning, suffering and*   161
> *death, guilt and shame, reconciliation and forgiveness, freedom and responsibility, hope*   162
> *and despair, love and joy).*   163
> *   2. Value-based considerations and attitudes (e.g., what is most important for each per-*   164
> *son, such as relations to oneself, family, friends, work, aspects of nature, art and culture,*   165
> *ethics and morals, and life itself).*   166
> *   3. Religious considerations and foundations (e.g., faith, beliefs and practices, the rela-*   167
> *tionship with God or the ultimate).*   168

2.3 Being a Human Being   169

Spirituality, as we suggested, is the experience of inevitable 'givens' or basic condi-   170
tions of human life. In other words, it is an 'anthropological structure' (a structural   171
aspect of being human). However, the question remains, what *is* it to be a human   172
being? This is a very significant question, and many approaches have strived to   173
develop answers, including the role of spirituality in our lives. In this section, we   174
will investigate this a little further and consider the relevance of spiritual care in   175
healthcare.   176

2.3.1 The Lived Body   177

One way of approaching what it is to be a human being is to note that being human   178
is always to find oneself in an embodied existence. To highlight this, a French phi-   179
losopher, Maurice Merleau-Ponty, developed his concept of the 'Lived Body' [12].   180
This notion is based on an understanding of the human being as relational and inte-   181
grated with their environment. Merleau-Ponty suggested that a human being is an   182
embodied self who stands in a sensory interaction within the world. Merleau-   183
Ponty's thesis focuses on the world only being accessible to humans through our   184

185 senses. In other words, the senses are our main prerequisite for understanding the
186 world in which we live. Merleau-Ponty argues that a human is not (only) in the
187 world as a thinking consciousness, as some of the modern philosophers suggest, but
188 also as a body—a lived body—that is both subject and object, seeing and seen, sens-
189 ing and sensed, touching and touched, moving and moved [13].

190   Someone who has elaborated on Merleau-Ponty's notion of the lived body in a
191 healthcare setting, is the medical doctor and professor, Anna Luise Kirkengen [14].
192 Her research focuses on, among other things, the 'inscribed body' and health impact
193 on sexual abuse in childhood [15, 16]. The body carries the effect of living life as it
194 is experienced in interaction with its surroundings [17, 18]. Kirkengen emphasises
195 that the sensory perception and cognitive awareness are joined to a specific mean-
196 ing, self-perceived actions and self-referencing experiences. Together they consti-
197 tute a very special *lived meaning*. This encompasses the lived body (the body's lived
198 time) along with the rooms and places you have lived in and the relationships you
199 have had. In other words, the concept of lived meaning opens up the world of per-
200 ceptions and memories that every human being has and is being shaped by, and
201 therefore, the body is incorporated with experiences [14].

202   Consequently, the body is seen as a carrier of the human being's history, with our
203 thoughts not without a body, and our emotions having the body as a precondition.
204 We cannot know, feel, learn and experience anything without the body being
205 involved. Therefore, it becomes pointless to talk about, for instance, 'purely mental'
206 trauma. The human spiritual, mental and physical aspects belong together.

207   This means that the perspectives on 'the lived body' involve a critique of tradi-
208 tional biomedical thinking, which tends to reduce human existence to the physical.
209 According to Kirkengen [16], the production of traditional biomedical knowledge
210 has not focused sufficiently on understanding how experiences related to self-image,
211 relationships and values are 'inscribed' in the body ([19], p. 683). She therefore
212 argues for a paradigm shift within the medical tradition that has long divided people
213 experiencing illness into somatic and psychological categories. Instead, she believes
214 that we need a professional language that makes it possible to conceptualise body
215 and mind as *undivided and integrated* [19]. Essentially, the lived body *always* inter-
216 acts with three phenomena: body, experience and meaning.

217   As already mentioned, the human spiritual, mental and physical aspects have
218 been distinguished, but belong together. This interdependence between body, mind
219 and spirit is acutely realised at times when different spiritual stressors can invariably
220 lead to increasing one's vulnerability for illness and disease, and vice versa.
221 Moreover, experienced support, acknowledgement and belonging can contribute to
222 strengthen the health condition [19].

2.3.2   Basic Conditions for Human Life

224 As we suggested, human life is not whatever we choose it to be, but to one degree
225 or another, it has certain 'basic conditions' we are inevitably faced with. These con-
226 ditions refer to five givens we cannot 'choose away' from our lives [20, 21]. The

first condition is that we all are vulnerable. We can be hurt in many ways, for 227
instance, emotionally, spiritually and physically. In the framework of the lived body, 228
being hurt in one of these dimensions cannot be separated from the other parts, 229
because every part is linked to the others. A second condition is that people are 230
interdependent on each other. We need others and others need us, so what other 231
people do may influence (either directly or indirectly) our lives. A third condition is 232
that people inevitably make mistakes and therefore relationships can be fragile. The 233
fourth condition is that life has a definitive end and we are limited by death. Finally, 234
the fifth condition regards being cared for by others, because we cannot live without 235
each other's care and support. In particular, we need each other's care when we are 236
in more vulnerable situations, during childhood. 237

There are many ways of trying to say something about what it is to be a human 238
being. The moment of birth is a time of grace in which connections with others 239
(either present in person or not) across professional boundaries, places of birth and 240
types of birth were transcended [22]. The notion of the 'lived body'; that all our 241
experiences are dimensions of the body, and that spiritual, mental and physical 242
aspects belong together in our embodied existence, helps us to see some important 243
aspects of what it can be to be a human being. Moreover, this lived body with its 244
basic conditions for human life provides a conceptual framework for understanding 245
the relevance of *being* human in the provision of spiritual care. 246

2.4 Spiritual Care: What It Is and How to Do it?   247

After a theoretical section on spirituality, let us start the next section on spiritual 248
care with two stories from clinical practice. This will give us examples of what 249
spiritual care can be—and of what it should not be. After this practical exploration, 250
we can then move on to a more general description and discussion account the con- 251
cept of spiritual care. 252

Activity 3
Please read the scenario below and ask what this account tells you about the delivery of spiritual care?

Mr. C's mobility had been affected by his stroke. The likelihood of returning to his previous level of fitness was poor. A member of the therapy team noted that he had seemed despondent during a session and was concerned that he was struggling with something.

I went to see Mr. C and noticed he did indeed look reserved and troubled. I tried to start a conversation, but unsurprisingly I did not get very far when I asked if he felt OK or if anything was bothering him. I needed to find a way to connect with him.

> *I asked him about what he liked to do and when he said that he had been a keen hiker I was able to express my own enthusiasm and shared some of my experiences with him. We continued sharing stories for a while and any concerns I had about 'rubbing salt in the wound' [by making a painful experience even more painful for someone] were quickly gone as I saw him cheer up and become more excited by the memories of his adventures.*
>
> *We eventually touched upon an incredible moment. He described to me hiking in the Himalayas, so I asked him whether he had been near Mount Everest whilst he was there. Then, I watched as he was whisked away with his memory. He told me about the moment when he had come to the top of a valley, looked up and saw Everest shining in the sky. The Tibetans have strong spiritual ties with Everest and call her the goddess mother of the world.*
>
> *Just watching the expression on this man's face was enough to tell me that this had been a significant experience for him. He spoke about it with reverence, with a tear in his eye. It was so clear that this was more to him than just seeing a mountain.*

253   This scenario affirms that spirituality is concerned with how individuals find
254   meaning, purpose and fulfilment in life, and in this situation, it involved climbing
255   and being immersed in nature. It was clear that the nurse or healthcare professional
256   was able to develop a rapport and establish trust with the gentleman through their
257   shared and mutual interests.

Activity 4
Please can you read the following scenario and consider when spiritual care is absent or lacking in the delivery of care:

> *I visited a friend in hospital who was in the terminal phase of her disease. She was an anaesthesiologist, and she spent her entire working life at that hospital where she was currently admitted. She complained to me that her doctor had told her to prepare for a diagnostic test.*
>
> *When I told her that she should probably have additional diagnostics to help control her pain, she replied that everyone just kept talking about diagnostic tests and medication, and none of her colleagues had ever taken five minutes to sit next to her and talk to her about what lies ahead of her. She said she had a feeling they were treating her as a case to learn from.*
>
> *"I just want to talk about everyday things, what they prepared for lunch today, what they bought, and what kind of play they will see at the theatre. I would have been happier if they had simply brought me a book to read than prescribe a new therapy".*

Reflective Questions

Having read through the scenarios you may like to reflect upon the following questions?

1. *What was the main focus of care in these two situations?*
2. *What was missing from this caring interaction?*
3. *How might a focus on the spiritual aspect of the person have enhanced the quality of care provided?*

2.4.1 Spiritual Care: Theoretical Perspectives

Spirituality is a trait of every human individual and therefore a subjective experience. In an ideal world, spiritual care in nursing and midwifery would be established and guided and based on every model or theory of clinical practice. Martsolf and Mickley [23] provide a very useful overview of the extent that spirituality is addressed within nursing models. Fortunately, because of the developments in nursing, there are many theories of nursing and midwifery. We name just a few.

Florence Nightingale's theory is based on the belief that acting for the benefit of others is the primary way of serving God. The foundation of care is defined as a religious calling [24]. She believed that health care should serve the search for truth, i.e., the discovery of God's laws of healing, and their proper application [25].

Therapist, Margaret Jean Harman Watson, defined nursing as a set of attitudes based on knowledge and commitment to the work of caring [26]. A nurse is a person who knows the individual person, healthy or sick, and who promotes this person's health. Watson describes a person as a human being with a psychological and physical, but above all, a spiritual longing for the accomplishment of spiritual 'quests' in life. When defining a person, Watson refers to the dependence between the patient and the nurse who complement each other in the caring relationship. In her profound descriptions, Watson often defines illness as an imbalance of spirituality, body and mind, including spiritual care as part of addressing the illness of a human being [26]. The essential phenomenon of the nursing theory is caring for an individual person as the fundamental task and ideal of nursing [27].

Joyce Travelbee noted in her theory of illness as a 'self-actualizing experience' [28] that a person's spiritual values determine one's personal perception of illness. The nurse's philosophical beliefs and spiritual values will determine the degree to which they will assist the patient in finding meaning of life.

Betty Neuman's conceptual model describes spirituality as an innate variable of an individual that affects health and stability [29]. Because a person's health, ability to prevent illness and cope with illness depend on the interrelatedness of the spiritual, social, physical and mental developmental variables of human functioning, addressing the spiritual aspect of health and illness is an integral part of nursing care.

290   Since spirituality is a dimension of being human, and being human means being
291   vulnerable, suffering, mortal and so on, disease and illness have a spiritual dimen-
292   sion. To facilitate care for a patient, and not in the least to honour their dignity as a
293   human being, care for the patient's spiritual experience of being ill and being cared
294   for is an integral part of the nurse's and midwife's professional role. To be sure, the
295   nurse's or midwife's own spiritual values, life experience, and professional beliefs
296   about illness and suffering determine the degree to which the nurse or midwife is
297   prepared and able to assist patients in discovering and maintaining spirituality. All
298   persons are valued as spiritual beings, meaning human beings with a spiritual
299   dimension.
300   A person may be spiritual but not clearly in a specific religious sense. They may
301   not belong to a particular religious tradition or community, nor think, speak or act
302   in the language of a specific religion. If we go back in European history, spirituality
303   is a Christian concept described as early as the fifth century. Today, the word 'spiri-
304   tuality' is sometimes understood in the vein of esoteric, Eastern religions, or so-
305   called new religions or new modern 'self-realising' movements. Still, historically
306   speaking, 'piety' was the proper term for spirituality. Especially in Christian theol-
307   ogy the spirituality and piety are still used as synonyms [4].
308   Due to the advancement of the medical sciences on the one hand, and the dehu-
309   manisation of health care on the other, the success of treating patients is often
310   equated with the ability to use the latest medical technologies, while forgetting the
311   dignity of the patient. In contacts with the patient, health care is often focused on the
312   symptoms, on the relief of physical pain and often not allowed the time to listen to
313   the patient's thoughts and struggles. In this technical environment, women may be
314   deprived of celebration of their uniqueness and power during the childbirth experi-
315   ence; thus, opportunities for enhancing and embracing the potentially spiritual
316   experience of birth are compromised [30]. However, in addition to medication and
317   so on, a patient needs the presence of another kind: spiritual help and support.
318   Nurses and midwives whose spiritual care for the patient include openness, compas-
319   sion, warmth, understanding, and support most often take up this role.
320   The EPICC network has in the EPICC Spiritual Care Education Standard agreed
321   to use the following description, saying that spiritual care means:

322   *Care which recognises and responds to the human spirit when faced with life-changing*
323   *events (such as birth, trauma, ill health, loss) or sadness, and can include the need for*
324   *meaning, for self-worth, to express oneself, for faith support, perhaps for rites or prayer or*
325   *sacrament, or simply for a sensitive listener. Spiritual care begins with encouraging human*
326   *contact in compassionate relationship and moves in whatever direction need requires.*
327   *([31] p. 6)*

2.4.2   Meeting Spiritual Needs in Time of Vulnerability

329   The need for spiritual care in supporting openings for meaning in life is emphasised
330   most often when nurses and midwives deal with challenging situations such as com-
331   plicated birth, serious illness and end-of-life care. It is the nurse or midwife who is

usually present with the patient, keeps track of the condition and has knowledge and skills for reading verbal and non-verbal communication regarding a patient's needs. Meeting spiritual needs is typically very important for the patient. Spiritual well-being means that the patient has a lower degree of anxiety, tolerates pain more easily, goes through the stages of birth or illness more calmly and welcomes the creation of a new life or the end of life when ready.

Spirituality is the sense of uniqueness, identity and worth to the patient and works as an internal source of strength. Taking care of spiritual needs, the nurse and midwife provides support to the patient and their family in a non-judgmental way, while understanding, accepting and reconciling with others and life itself. Spiritual care, in the sense of 'being with' the patient, can involve the nurse or midwife being compassionate, caring, supportive and perhaps offering prayer. Fundamentally, being near the patient, and 'walking' with them, even in silence, can have a greater effect than words because spiritual pain is not a problem that needs to be resolved. These are aspects of care that will be revisited throughout the following chapters of this book.

2.5 Spiritual Care: Some Examples from Across Europe

2.5.1 Spiritual Care in the Netherlands

In the second half of the twentieth century, secularisation has spread in the Netherlands. By the beginning of the twenty-first century, less than half of the population associate themselves with traditional religions. The group of theists, those who believe in a God, have decreased from 50% to 15% of the population. Still, a group of 75% can be called 'spiritual' in some way or another, i.e., they are aware of existential questions and practices that relates to existential meaning. Spirituality and religion have become much more individualised. It is still relevant, but it has new faces.

In the Netherlands, a new definition of health becomes influential. The World Health Organization [32] defines health not only as the absence of disease or infirmity but a state of complete physical, mental and social well-being. However, many people in our society must deal with diseases without the prospect of their absence, such as when people live with chronic/long-term conditions and increasing health conditions in older people. From that perspective, Huber et al. [33] proposed a new definition of so-called positive health, being: 'the ability to adapt and to self-manage, in the face of social, physical and emotional challenges' (p. 1). This definition makes daily functioning, resilience and self-direction of the patient more central than the treatment of disease. In this model of positive health, spirituality/meaning is one of the dimensions of health.

This illustrates how spirituality is resurfacing as a dimension of health care in the Netherlands. Some of the current topics in Dutch health care related to spirituality are end-of-life questions, issues about over-treatment of diseases, dignity in care for

372 older people, palliative care, the psychosocial approach of dementia and mental
373 health recovery. Traditional chaplaincy is changing. Healthcare workers such as
374 nurses and midwifes, too, now must address these spiritual challenges.
375   Therefore, new developments are taking place in health care in the Netherlands.
376 Projects to implement multidisciplinary spiritual care in community care and to
377 strengthen the professional role of chaplaincy are sponsored by the government. In
378 palliative care, a multidisciplinary guideline about spiritual care is developed and
379 implemented in practice. In mental health care, a similar guideline is under con-
380 struction. Initiatives are taken to embed spiritual care in curricula (medicine, nurs-
381 ing and social work). Specific tools are designed for spiritual care in practice (e.g.,
382 assessment and referral) and in education (e.g., online tools). Research in spiritual
383 care and professional support is more practice oriented and focussed on develop-
384 ment of best practices.

385 ## 2.5.2 Spiritual Care in Croatia

386 When talking to students and nurses about spirituality and providing spiritual
387 care in health care, they first think of religion. Spirituality is understood as faith
388 in a relationship with God; it brings peace, prosperity, joy, security, kindness,
389 patience and love into human life. Faith as part of spirituality maintains the mean-
390 ing of life during pain and suffering. Health care helps a patient in his illness to
391 find hope, comfort and inner peace in everyday life as well as to find meaning
392 in life.
393   The word spirituality does not yet have an exact definition in the culture of living
394 of the Croatian people; the term religiosity is more appropriate. Religion is a belief
395 system by which one enters the relationship with God and secures salvation. When
396 we talk about spirituality, we can be in a relationship with prayer and God, but also
397 with nature, friends, things, events.
398   In the Croatian language, the term 'religion' is different from the term 'religios-
399 ity'. Religion means institutions, system, something structural and common.
400 Religiosity is individual and subjective, refers to experience, relation to God and
401 can be understood as creating a connection with the transcendental. The different
402 dimensions of religiosity are often not interconnected and are an indicator that reli-
403 giosity is a multidimensional construct.
404   The perception of the term 'spiritual well-being' opens the picture of wholeness
405 versus fragmentation, and as a proof of spiritual well-being, there is self-respect,
406 selfless giving, moral character, belief in the omnipresent God and personal tran-
407 scendence. Although religiosity and spirituality have different concepts, they are
408 nevertheless linked. Some definitions and measurements of spirituality require the
409 separation of religiosity and spirituality, which is very important to persons who are
410 considered spiritual and not religious.

2.5.3 Spiritual Care in Norway

₄₁₁

Norway is regarded to be one of the most secular countries in the world. Still, approximately 70% of the population are members of the Norwegian Lutheran church, but church attendance is low at about 2%. Nevertheless, many people choose to participate during rituals in the church, as baptism, weddings and funerals. About 25% of the population view themselves as non-religious and do not believe in God or other higher powers and have no everyday rituals related to religion [34]. Empirical research of Norwegian citizens' own view on health showed surprising findings [35]. Most of the informants reported that to believe in God could be a health asset. Religion as a health asset was in particular viewed as important in crises, providing sources for coping and quality of life. Religion was also described to be important for preventing feelings of guilt and for accepting the human being as fallible and imperfect. As an overall finding, religion was perceived as a counterculture to perfection, providing fellowship, relations and meaning.

In the education of nursing and midwifery students, holistic care is emphasised. The concept of 'spiritual care' has been used as a part of holistic care. However, the concept 'spiritual' has some downsides in the Norwegian context. For instance, the concept is difficult to define, and people's spirituality is regarded to be private. Spirituality also has a connotation to religion, which does not correspond well to a secular view of life. In this context, the use of the concept 'existential' gained prominence. The existential relates to the structures of *being* a human being and to questions like 'what is the meaning, value and purpose of life and death'? The concept can be closely linked to the spiritual, but not necessarily spiritual per se [36]. Thus, the concept 'existential' is increasingly used in the Norwegian context.

2.5.4 Summary of European Examples

₄₃₆

While this section has outlined some developments and perspectives from within Europe, it must be stated that the concepts of spirituality and spiritual care are being explored internationally. The published literature would suggest that nurses, and to a lesser extent midwives, from every continent are engaging with these concepts and undertaking research in this field. This awareness is important because nursing and midwifery practice across the globe are undertaken within diverse cultural settings. Therefore, a one-size-fits-all approach is not appropriate. How nurses and midwives understand spirituality in the United States may be totally different to how this is perceived by nursing and midwives working in Asia. While there may be many commonalities in how these concepts are understood and practiced, assumptions and generalisations cannot be imposed, and sensitivity is required when discussing and exploring these concepts.

2.6 Summary

The aim of this chapter was to provide some reflections regarding the terms 'spirituality' and 'spiritual care'. We started with the observation that there is plenty of literature in nursing and midwifery offering numerous definitions of spirituality. This raised two questions. The first question was what is the phenomenon these definitions try to point to? The second question was what definition should be used in this book?

As an answer to the first question, we suggested that spirituality is an experience, namely the awareness of our 'human condition'. By this, we mean the 'inevitable givens' or 'basic conditions' of life. Furthermore, this experience and our practices of awareness usually accord with an evaluation of one's human condition. That is why we often talk about spirituality in terms of 'existential meaning'. These first two points: (1) spirituality as experience and (2) spirituality as experience of existential meaning, often relate to, for example, the birth experience, transition to motherhood, one's health and hence to the context of impaired life experiences, health and healthcare. This means that its presence in nursing and midwifery is inevitable. Lastly, it is of clinical relevance to note that these experiences (and practices) of spirituality are most often expressed in (parts of) religious language.

Given this broad phenomenon and variety of definitions, the EPICC project and its subsequent network reached consensus for a working definition developed by the European Association for Palliative Care (EAPC). Specifically, that spirituality is the dimension of human life that relates to the way persons' experience meaning and the way they connect to the world around them.

Spirituality is therefore an 'anthropological structure', i.e., a structural aspect of being human. However, the question remains of what it is to be a human being? One way of approaching this is to note that being human is always an embodied existence. The body carries the effects of living life as it is experienced in interaction with its surroundings. Consequently, the body is a carrier of the human being's history. In our professional language, we conceptualise body and mind as undivided and integrated. The living human being always interacts with body, experience and meaning. Physical, mental and spiritual aspects of the living body belong together. That means spiritual stressors can lead to vulnerability for illness and diseases, and vice versa.

What we call the anthropological structure of being human suggests five basic conditions relevant to nursing and midwifery. The first condition is that we all are vulnerable. A second condition is that people are interdependent on each other. A third condition is that people unavoidably make mistakes and therefore relationships are fragile. The fourth condition is that we are limited by death. Finally, the fifth condition concerning being cared-for by others because we cannot live without each other's care.

References

1. Puchalski C, Vitillo R, Hull S, Reller N. Improving the spiritual dimension of whole person care: reaching national and international consensus. J Palliat Med. 2014;17(6):642–56. https://doi.org/10.1089/jpm.2014.9427.
2. Nash DB, Yuen E. The role of spirituality in health. MedPage Today. 2009. https://www.medpagetoday.com/columns/focusonpolicy/14725. Accessed 12 Apr 2019.
3. Puchalski C, Ferrell B. Making healthcare whole: integrating spirituality into patient care. West Conshohocken, PA: Templeton Press; 2010.
4. Koenig HG, King DE, Carson VB. Handbook of religion and health. Oxford, NewYork: Oxford University Press; 2012.
5. Canfield C, et al. Critical care Nurses' perceived need for guidance in addressing spirituality in critically ill patients. Am J Crit Care. 2016;25(3):206–11.
6. Crowther S, Hall J. Spirituality and spiritual care in and around childbirth. Women Birth. 2015;28(2):173–8. https://doi.org/10.1016/j.wombi.2015.01.001.
7. Hay D. Something there the biology of the human Spirit. London: Darton Longman and Todd; 2006.
8. DeMarinis V. The impact of Postmodernization on existential health in Sweden: psychology of Religion's function in existential public health analysis. Arch Psychol Relig. 2008;30:57–74.
9. Baumiller R. Spiritual development during a first pregnancy. Int J Childbirth Educ. 2002;17:7.
10. Callister LC, Khalaf I. Spirituality in childbearing women. J Perinatal Educ. 2010;19(2):16–24.
11. European Association for Palliaitve Care. EAPC task force on spiritual care in palliative care. n.d. https://www.eapcnet.eu/eapc-groups/task-forces/spiritual-care. Accessed 18 Feb 2019.
12. Langer MM, Merleau-Ponty M. Merleau-Ponty's phenomenology of perception : a guide and commentary. London: Macmillan; 1989.
13. Merleau-Ponty M. Phenomenology of perception. Boca Raton, FL: Taylor and Francis; 2002.
14. Kirkengen AL. Hvordan krenkede barn blir syke voksne. 2nd ed. Oslo: Universitetsforl; 2009.
15. Kirkengen AL. Embodiment of sexual boundary violations in childhood: a phenomenological-hermeneutical study of the health impact of childhood sexual abuse. Oslo: Institute of General Practice and Community Medicine, Department of General Practice, University of Oslo; 1998.
16. Kirkengen AL. Inscribed bodies: health impact of childhood sexual abuse. Dordrecht: Kluwer; 2001.
17. Kirkengen AL, Shaw ES. The lived experience of violation: how abused children become unhealthy adults. Bucharest: Zeta Books; 2010.
18. Kirkengen AL. Creating chronicity. J Eval Clin Pract. 2017;23(5):1071–4. https://doi.org/10.1111/jep.12715.
19. Getz L, Kirkengen AL, Ulvestad E. The human biology—with experience. Tidsskr Nor Legeforen. 2011;131:683. https://doi.org/10.4045/tidsskr.10.0874.
20. Henriksen J-O, Vetlesen AJ. *Nærhet og distanse: grunnlag, verdier og etiske teorier i arbeid med mennesker* [proximity and distance: basis, values and ethical theories in working with people]. 3rd ed. Oslo: Gyldendal akademisk; 2006.
21. Macquarry J. In search of humanity. A theological and philosophical approach. London: SCM Press; 1982.
22. Crowther S. Sacred joy at birth: a hermeneutic phenomenology study. PhD, Auckland University of Technology. 2014. https://openrepository.aut.ac.nz/handle/10292/7071.
23. Martsolf DS, Mickley JR. The concept of spirituality in nursing theories: differing world views and extent of focus. J Adv Nurs. 1998;27:294–303.
24. Gonzalo A. Florence Nightingale's biography and environmental theory: study guide. 2019. https://nurseslabs.com/florence-nightingales-environmental-theory/. Accessed 11 Mar 2019.
25. Parker ME. Nursing theories & nursing practice. Philadelphia: F. A. Davis; 2005.
26. Watson J. Caring as the essence and science of nursing and health care. Caring. 1999;48(6):288–98.
27. Tomey AM, Alligood MR. Nursing theorists and their work. St. Louis: Mosby; 2002.

542 28. O'Brien ME. Spirituality in nursing: standing on holy ground. 6th ed. Burlington, MA: Jones
543   & Bartlett Learning; 2017.
544 29. Reed KS. Betty Neuman: The Neuman Systems Model (notes on nursing theories), vol. 11.
545   London: Sage; 1993.
546 30. Davis-Floyd RE. Birth as an American rite of passage. 2nd ed. London: University of California
547   Press; 2003.
548 31. NHS Scotland. Spiritual care matters: an introductory resource for all NHS Scotland staff.
549   2010. https://www.nes.scot.nhs.uk/media/3723/spiritualcaremattersfinal.pdf. Accessed 18
550   Feb 2019.
551 32. World Health Organization (WHO). Constitution. Geneva: WHO; 1948.
552 33. Huber M, van Vliet M, Giezenberg M, Winkens B, Heerkens Y, Dagnelie PC, Knottnerus
553   JA. Towards a 'patient-centred' operationalisation of the new dynamic concept of health: a mixed
554   methods study. BMJ Open. 2016;5:e010091. https://doi.org/10.1136/bmjopen-2015-010091.
555 34. Skålvoll Urstad S. De fleste ikke-religiøse er medlemmer av kirken. [Most non-religious are members
556   of the Church] Forskning. no. 2018. https://forskning.no/religion-universitetet-i-agder-partner/
557   de-fleste-ikke-religiose-er-medlemmer-av-kirken/1223089.
558 35. Fugelli P, Ingstad B. Helse på norsk: god helse slik folk ser det; 2009.
559 36. Lundmark M. Religiös och icke-religiös andlighet. In: Friberg IF, Öhlén J, editors.
560   Omvårdnadens grunder. Perspektiv och förhållningssätt. Lund: Studentlitteratur AB; 2019.
561   p. 509–37.

Suggested Reading

563 Balthip S, McSherry W, Kittikorn N. Spirituality and dignity of Thai adolescents living with
564   HIV. Religions. 2017;8(257):1–18. https://doi.org/10.3390/rel8120257.
565 Niu Y, McSherry W, Partridge M. The perceptions of spirituality and spiritual care among people
566   from Chinese backgrounds living in England: a grounded theory method. J Transcult Nurs.
567   2020. https://doi.org/10.1177/1043659620938135

Chapter 3
Educational Context, Evidence and Exploration of Professional Fields of Nursing and Midwifery

Linda Ross, Janet Holt, Britt Moene Kuven, Birthe Ørskov, and Piret Paal

Learning Objectives

This chapter will enable you to:

1. Identify who is calling for nurses/midwives to be competent in spiritual care, namely (1) healthcare policymakers, (2) nursing and midwifery professional/regulatory bodies, (3) patients and carers, (4) nurses and midwives.
2. Reflect on what this may mean for your practice using case studies and reflective exercises.
3. Identify how the EPICC Project has responded to this call.

L. Ross (✉)
Faculty of Life Sciences and Education, School of Care Sciences, University of South Wales, Pontypridd, UK
e-mail: linda.ross@southwales.ac.uk

J. Holt
Royal College of Nursing UK Representative to EPICC, School of Healthcare, University of Leeds, Leeds, UK

B. M. Kuven
Department of Health and Caring Sciences, Western Norway University of Applied Sciences, Bergen, Norway

B. Ørskov
Faculty of Health, VID Specialized University, Bergen, Norway

The Deaconess University College, Nursing Education, Frederiksberg, Denmark

P. Paal
WHO Collaborating Centre, Institute for Nursing Science and Practice, Paracelsus Medical University, Salzburg, Austria

© Springer Nature Switzerland AG 2021
W. McSherry et al. (eds.), *Enhancing Nurses' and Midwives' Competence in Providing Spiritual Care*, https://doi.org/10.1007/978-3-030-65888-5_3

3.1   Introduction

This chapter will set the scene for the chapters that follow. Drawing upon international evidence, this chapter will explore the need for nurses and midwives to be
competent in spiritual care to meet expectations of international healthcare policy,
nursing and midwifery regulatory and professional bodies, and patients and carers.
Evidence suggests that nurses and midwives feel unprepared for their role in spiritual care, and they have called for more education. The EPICC Project has responded
to this call. Reflective exercises and case studies are provided throughout the chapter to engage the reader, whether they be a student, educator, practitioner, researcher,
manager or policymaker.

3.2   International Healthcare Policy

Healthcare policy internationally acknowledges the importance of the spiritual
dimension of people's lives for their health and well-being; however, varying terminology may be used including terms such as spiritual, religious, cultural, existential,
values and uniqueness of the individual.

3.2.1   *Internationally*

In 1946, the World Health Organization (WHO) considered but decided not to
include spiritual well-being in its definition of health: 'Health is a state of complete
physical, mental and social well-being and not merely the absence of disease or
infirmity' (WHO [online] Available at: https://www.who.int/about/who-we-are/
constitution# [Accessed 30/3/20]). However, spirituality has continued to be of
interest to the organisation. In 1984, the World Health Assembly (WHA) resolution
37.13 made the spiritual dimension part and parcel of WHO Member States' strategies for health [1]. In 1991, it acknowledged the importance of spirituality for peoples' lives, defining the spiritual dimension as:

> ...a phenomenon that is not material in nature, but belongs to the realm of ideas, beliefs,
> values and ethics that have arisen in the minds and conscience of human beings, particu-
> larly ennobling ideas. [...] The spiritual dimension plays a great role in motivating people's
> achievement in all aspects of life. [2]

In 1998, WHO acknowledged the limitations of the medical model. It considered
the model's '..mechanistic view of patients as being only a material body' as 'no
longer satisfactory'. It recognised the importance of 'spiritual elements' such as

'faith, hope and compassion in the healing process' and called for research to 'move towards a more holistic view of health that includes a non-material dimension' [3]. In 2002 the WHO endorsed spirituality as a health-related quality-of-life indicator [4].

3.2.2   Within Europe

The European Commission acknowledges 'spiritual' and 'cultural' aspects of life as important for healthy ageing and recommends that healthcare services provide person-centred care:

> Patient and their family rights include the right to….be treated with respect and care; have cultural practices and spiritual beliefs respected; and to be free from discrimination based on race, religion, culture, or gender. [5]

The Equality and Human Rights Commission [6] states that 'governments should provide for the spiritual and religious needs of their citizens', at the same time listing circumstances when being treated differently due to religion or belief is lawful.

3.2.3   Nationally

The Scottish Government was one of the first governments to require all healthcare providers in the country to develop and implement spiritual care policies and plans to meet the spiritual needs of the local population [7]. Other governments have since followed. For example, in 2009, the Norwegian Ministry of Health and Care Services published a White Paper stating that people dependent on municipal health and care services should be able to safeguard their opportunities for belief and practice of life (https://www.regjeringen.no/no/dokumenter/i-62009-rett-til-egen-tros%2D%2Dog-livssynsu/id587577/). This paper emphasised that health and care services are responsible for designing care services to take account of peoples' cultural and spiritual needs and personal preferences. The paper is supported with guidance, emphasising that the spiritual dimension is relevant for everyone and encompasses what is important to individuals, such as their identity, dreams, hope, values, faith and outlook on life. Denmark adopts a similar stance (https://www.sst.dk/da/sygdom-og-behandling/~/media/79CB83AB4DF74C80837BAAAD55347D0D.ashx). In Wales, person-centred care, which considers peoples 'spiritual, pastoral and religious' needs, is at the heart of the Welsh Government's Health and Care Standards [8].

70 *3.2.4 Spiritual Care Guidelines*

71 For healthcare providers in many countries, catering for the spiritual, religious and
72 pastoral needs of patients, carers and staff is important enough for them to employ
73 specialist spiritual care providers whose role is shaped by specific spiritual care
74 guidelines and competencies. For example, NHS England's Chaplaincy Guidelines
75 [9] and the UK Board of Healthcare Chaplaincy Standards for Healthcare
76 Chaplaincy [10].
77   However, spiritual care has probably received greatest attention within pal-
78 liative care through the hospice movement and its founder's, Dame Cicely
79 Saunders, notion of 'total pain', the suffering that encompasses all of a person's
80 physical, psychological, social, spiritual and practical struggles. Saunders con-
81 sidered the 'spiritual' to be about a person's moral values and spiritual pain was
82 a desolate sense of meaninglessness encountered by someone at the end of life.
83 Spirituality continues to be a core feature of most palliative care organisation,
84 for example guidelines produced by the European Association of Palliative Care
85 (EAPC), Marie Curie, Worldwide Hospice Palliative Care Alliance (WHPC).
86 The EAPC [11] provides the following definition reached through international
87 consensus:

88   *Spirituality is the dynamic dimension of human life that relates to the way persons (indi-*
89   *vidual and community) experience, express and/or seek meaning, purpose and transcen-*
90   *dence, and the way they connect to the moment, to self, to others, to nature, to the significant*
91   *and/or the sacred. The spiritual field is multidimensional, containing:*
92   *1. Existential challenges (e.g. questions concerning identity, meaning, suffering and*
93   *death, guilt and shame, reconciliation and forgiveness, freedom and responsibility, hope*
94   *and despair, love and joy).*
95   *2. Value based considerations and attitudes (what is most important for each person,*
96   *such as relations to oneself, family, friends, work, things, nature, art and culture, ethics and*
97   *morals, and life itself).*
98   *3. Religious considerations and foundations (faith, beliefs and practices, the relation-*
99   *ship with God or the ultimate.*

100 Most recently, a new EAPC white paper provides best practice guidelines for
101 educating palliative care staff to provide spiritual care [12]. While most spiritual
102 care guidelines stem from palliative care, others are starting to extend beyond that
103 to ageing and dementia care. Examples are outlined in Table 3.1.

104 *3.2.5 Spiritual Care Guidance for Nurses*

105 Spiritual care guidance is available for different professions, such as for psychia-
106 trists [13], but the focus of this chapter is on guidance for nurses and midwives who
107 have historically worked alongside other professionals, such as chaplains, in

Table 3.1 Examples of spiritual care guidelines

Country	Guideline
Palliative care	
Netherlands, translated into German, English and Spanish	Spiritual care guideline for multidisciplinary palliative care http://vivereilmorire.eu/wp-content/uploads/2017/09/Spiritual-care.pdf
Germany	Spiritual care guideline for non-clerical professions. Gratz M, Roser T. Spiritual Care in Qualifzierungskursen für nicht-seelsorgliche Berufe: Grundsätze der Deutschen Gesellschaft für Palliativmedizin (Münchner Reihe Palliative Care, Band 15) Kohlhammer: Stuttgart 2019. 98. DGP Position Paper Spiritual Care in Palliative Care (DGP 2007) Spirituelle Begleitung in der Palliativversorgung (2007), http://www.dgpalliativmedizin.de/images/stories/pdf/fachkompetenz/070709%20Spirituelle%20Begl%20in%20Pm%20070510.pdf
Switzerland	Guideline for inter-professional spiritual care in palliative care. Peng-Keller S et al. (2018) Spiritual Care in Palliative Care. Leitlinien zur interprofessionellen Praxis, Bern 2018. Online abrufbar unter:
Norway	Palliative care guidelines focusing on meeting the physical, mental, social and spiritual/existential needs of seriously ill and dying patients. Spirituality has three domains: (a) existential challenges and approaches, (b) value-based judgements and attitudes and (c) religious considerations and anchors. NOU 2017:15 På liv og død. Palliasjon til alvorlig syke og døende. On life and death. Palliation for the seriously ill and dying Oslo: Ministry of Health and Care Services, white paper on the management of the Ministry of Health and Care Services. Nasjonalt handlingsprogram for palliasjon i kreftomsorgen 03/15. National Professional Ministry of Health and Care Services Guidelines for Palliation in Norway Oslo: Helsedirektoratet 2015, white paper on the management of the Ministry of Health and Care Services
Spain	Spiritual care guidelines for clinicians working in palliative care. E. Benito, J. Barbero, M. Dones (2014) Espiritualidad en Clínica Una propuesta de evaluación y acompañamiento espiritual en Cuidados Paliativos. Monografías SECPAL, Madrid
Denmark	Department of Health spiritual care guidelines for palliative care in primary care, hospital and hospice settings https://www.sst.dk/da/udgivelser/2017/anbefalinger-for-den-palliative-indsats

(continued)

Table 3.1 (continued)

	Country	Guideline
t1.30 t1.31	UK	National Institute for Health & Care Excellence palliative/end of life care documents where spiritual care features (https://www.nice.org.uk/)
t1.32	*Older person/dementia care*	
t1.33 t1.34 t1.35 t1.36	Australia	National Guidelines for Spiritual Care in Aged Care to 'promote each consumer's emotional, spiritual and psychological well-being' *Meaningful Ageing Australia, (2016). National Guidelines for Spiritual Care in Aged Care. Meaningful Ageing Australia, Parkville*
t1.37 t1.38 t1.39 t1.40 t1.41 t1.42 t1.43 t1.44 t1.45	Norway	Parliamentary white papers stressing the importance of existential and spiritual needs for older people and for those with dementia. Health and care services in Norway focus on ensuring that the individual's beliefs and vision are discussed by health professionals caring for them. The authorities are keen to see spiritual and existential needs properly mapped out and addressed in a similar way to other health needs *Meld. St. 15 (2017–2018). Leve hele livet. En kvalitetsreform for eldre. Live all your life. A quality reform for the elderly. Oslo: Ministry of Health and Care Services* *Ministry of Health and Care Services, 2018, white paper on the management of the Health and Care Services* *Ministry of Health and Care Services. Nasjonale faglige retningslinje om demens. National professional guidelines on dementia. IS-2658. Ministry of Health and Care Services Oslo., 2017, white paper on the management of the Ministry of Health and Care Services*
t1.46 t1.47	Denmark	The National Knowledge Center for older and people with dementia has developed an education course in spiritual care: 2020. http://www.videnscenterfordemens.dk/kurser/2020/11/aandelig-og-eksistentiel-omsorg/

Table 3.2 Examples of spiritual care guidance for nurses and midwives   t2.1

Organisation	Guidance	
North American Nursing Diagnosis Association guidelines (NANDA)	In 1996, spiritual suffering and distress were included in the NANDA Nursing Diagnosis List. NANDA is a professional nursing organisation established to standardise terminology http://www.nandanursingdiagnosislist.org/functional-health-patterns/spiritual-suffering/	t2.3 t2.4 t2.5 t2.6 t2.7
Government of Canada 2012	Clinical Practice Guidelines for Nurses in Primary Care refers to spirituality in the adult mental health section where mental health is seen as a balance between mental, emotional, physical and spiritual health. Spiritual well-being is considered important for mental well-being that can be endangered by spiritual abuse or lack of religious/spiritual connection. Strong spirituality and/or cultural ties are listed as protective factors *Government of Canada 2012. Clinical Practice Guidelines for Nurses in Primary Care. Adult Care - Chapter 15 - Mental Health, https://www. canada.ca/en/indigenous-services-canada/services/first-nations-inuit--health/health-care-services/nursing/clinical-practice-guidelines-nurses-primary-care.html*	t2.8 t2.9 t2.10 t2.11 t2.12 t2.13 t2.14 t2.15 t2.16 t2.17 t2.18
National Health & Medical Research Council Australia	The Australian Clinical Practice Guideline states that 'religion may play a fundamental role in the person's attitude toward their disease and treatment. Spiritual support from their religious group may be important'. Thus, to provide end-of-life support, nurses are to 'enquire about spiritual needs and offer referral for pastoral care, if desired' *NHMRC 2003. Clinical practice guidelines for the psychosocial care of adults with cancer. https://canceraustralia.gov.au/sites/default/files/publications/pca-1-clinical-practice-guidelines-for-psychosocial-care-of--adults-with-cancer_504af02682bdf.pdf Accessed 12/3/20*	t2.19 t2.20 t2.21 t2.22 t2.23 t2.24 t2.25 t2.26 t2.27
Slovenian Association of Nurses and Midwives	Slovenia has produced a spiritual care guideline for nurses entitled 'General recommendations for spiritual care in nursing' (2019) *Andreja Mihelič Zajec, Igor Karnjuš, Katarina Babnik, Branko Klun in Klelija Štrancar (2019) Splošna priporočila za duhovno oskrbo v zdravstveni negi. Zbornica zdravstvene in babiške nege Slovenije – Zveza strokovnih društev medicinskih sester, babic in zdravstvenih tehnikov Slovenije. Ljubljana, Slovenia*	t2.28 t2.29 t2.30 t2.31 t2.32 t2.33 t2.34
Royal College of Nursing of the United Kingdom (RCN)	The RCN produced guidance for nurses in the form of the 'spirituality in nursing care: a pocket guide' in response to a survey in which members said they felt unprepared for spiritual care *(https://www.rcn.org.uk/professional-development/publications/pub-003861) Accessed 19/3/20 http://www.elament.org.uk/media/1205/spirituality_in_nursing_care-_rcn_pocket_guide.pdf Accessed 12/3/20*	t2.35 t2.36 t2.37 t2.38 t2.39 t2.40

providing spiritual care as part of their holistic caring role. Table 3.2 gives examples   108
of spiritual care guidelines for nurses and midwives, and Box 3.1 offers an opportu-   109
nity to reflect on this.   110

Box 3.1: Reflection Exercise 1
1. Does your local health policy say anything about spiritual care? If yes, what terminology is used? Is it helpful to you in your practice? If not, do you think it should include spiritual care?

2. Do you know of any spiritual care guidance where you work, like the examples outlined in Table 3.2? This may have been produced by chaplains, nurses or an organisation. Look at the guidance. What do you think about it? Is it helpful?

3.3 Nursing and Midwifery Regulatory and Professional Bodies

Nursing and midwifery statutory bodies are usually established by a government to regulate the profession. For example, the Nursing and Midwifery Council (NMC) in the UK has a duty to protect the public. In pursuit of this, its functions include setting standards of education, training, conduct and performance, ensuring nurses and midwives keep their skills and knowledge up to date and uphold the NMC's professional standards. They also have a regulatory function in maintaining a register of nurses and midwives, with processes to investigate those who fall short of the professional standards. The functions of a statutory or regulatory body differ from those of a professional body, such as the International Council of Nurses (ICN), The Danish Nurses Organisation, The Norwegian Nurses Association, or the Royal Colleges in the UK. These organisations support nurses in a variety of ways including employment rights and education, but unlike a statutory or regulatory body, they have no authority over professional standards or those for education and training.

The NMC considers prioritising people as a key feature of nursing and midwifery practice and requires practitioners to recognise diversity and individual choice. But despite referring to physical social and psychological needs, spiritual needs are not identified specifically in its key document, the NMC Code [14]. In 2018 the NMC published new standards both for student education and for registered nurses; the latter consisting of proficiencies grouped together under seven platforms reflecting what a newly registered nurse should know and be capable of doing safely and proficiently at the start of their career [15]. In platform three of the proficiencies which addresses assessing needs and planning care, the NMC makes specific reference to spirituality, '*Registered nurses prioritise the needs of people when assessing and reviewing their mental, physical, cognitive, behavioural, social and spiritual needs*' ([15], p. 13).

In the introduction to the new Standards of Proficiency for Midwives, published by the NMC in 2019, reference is made to midwives supporting '*safe physical, psychological, social, cultural and spiritual situations*' (p. 4), and spirituality, spiritual situations, spiritual factors and spiritual safety are identified in three of the six domains into which the standards of proficiency are grouped [16]. While the Standards for Preregistration Midwifery Programmes [17] identifies spiritual factors equally with physical, psychological, social and cultural factors, this is not replicated in the Standards for Preregistration Nursing programmes. Also, the overarching Standards Framework for Nursing and Midwifery Education [18] is not specific about any curriculum content including spirituality, this being left up to each educational institution to decide. Hence, there is the potential for a lack of parity in spirituality education for nursing and midwifery students across the UK. How much teaching occurs is likely to be dependent on the weight an institution places on spirituality in comparison to other subjects. Interestingly an international survey of 2193 nursing students across eight European countries found that students identified caring for patients was the most influencing factor in their learning about spiritual care. The findings of this study highlight where theoretical knowledge is placed in the curriculum and a link between practice and university-based learning may be of importance [19].

The ICN, a federation of over 130 nursing associations, aims to represent nursing worldwide, advance the profession, promote well-being for nurses and be a health advocate. The Council has a Code of Ethics published in 2012 which specifically refers to spiritual beliefs as an important aspect of nursing care along with respect for human rights, values and customs. However, there does not appear to be any further comment or guidance from the ICN on standards for spirituality in nursing education. While the Council has broad international membership, its status is one of a professional rather than a statutory or regulatory body, and hence, its influence is restricted to being advisory rather than mandatory.

As a professional body in the UK, the Royal College of Nursing (RCN) supports nurses in continuing and professional education and promotes nursing research. Findings from a survey conducted by the RCN in 2010 revealed that respondents felt that guidance and support from professional, regulatory and statutory bodies was needed to ensure nurses could engage effectively in delivering spiritual care. This resulted in the publication of guidance 'Spirituality in Nursing Care: a pocket guide' (see Table 3.2) which is available for use by registered nurses and students.

Other European countries take different approaches to regulation of the profession and education programmes leading to registration of nurses and midwives. For example, in Denmark spiritual care has been integrated into the nursing curriculum following educational reform in 2001 (https://www.retsinformation.dk/pdfprint. aspx?id=114493). In Norway, new common guidelines for pre-registration undergraduate nursing degrees were produced by the Norwegian Ministry of Education and Research in 2019 (https://lovdata.no/dokument/SF/forskrift/2019-03-15-412). In these guidelines, the purpose of nurse education is that it should *'qualify candidates to practice nursing to attend to the basic needs of human beings, promote health, prevent and treat illness, relieve suffering and ensure a dignified death'*. Hence, the foundation for preparing practitioners to deliver caring and professionally sound nursing is up-to-date knowledge. Similar to the UK, the Norwegian regulations do not identify spiritual care as a separate learning outcome. But they do state that the student must have broad knowledge of the basic needs of the person, of the nurse's health-promoting, preventive, treating, rehabilitative and alleviating function, including knowledge of palliation. The student is also expected to have broad knowledge of person-centred nursing as well as insight into the Norwegian Nurses Organisations's Code of Ethics for Nurses.

Statutory and regulatory bodies expect nurses and midwives to recognise diversity, personal choice and spiritual needs of individuals in their care. However, there

193 is scant reference to spiritual care in curriculum requirements in education pro-
194 grammes leading to professional registration. The 'packed nursing curriculum' is
195 often cited as a reason; hence, education in spiritual care may not be seen as a prior-
196 ity by either educators or students in comparison to other competing subjects. Fear
197 of doing the wrong thing is another possible reason for spirituality not being
198 addressed in curricula. A case study example of this is provided in Box 3.2.
199 Professional bodies such as the ICN may be more explicit about the importance of
200 spiritual care in their documents, but this is unlikely to be recognised in any mean-
201 ingful way by nurse and midwifery educators without endorsement by a statutory or
202 regulatory body. In the UK, discussions have been on-going since 2015 with the
203 NMC about reinstating 'spiritual' within The Code [20, 21].

Box 3.2: Case Study

In 2008, Caroline Petrie a community nurse was suspended by her employer
North Somerset Primary Care Trust (PCT) for breaching the NMC Code by
using her professional status *to promote causes not related to health* and failing to *demonstrate a personal and professional commitment to equality and
diversity.* Ms. Petrie had offered to pray for a patient she visited, and while the
patient was not offended, she told another health worker what had happened,
and this ultimately led to her suspension.

1. The PCT cited the NMC Code in the reason for suspension. Do you think
   this is a correct interpretation of the Code? Which sections of the Code
   matched their accusations that Ms. Petrie:

   (a) Used her professional status to promote causes not related to health.
   (b) Failed to demonstrate a personal and professional commitment to
       equality and diversity.

2. Despite citing the NMC Code as the reason for Ms. Petrie's suspension,
   the NMC did not investigate her fitness to practice.

   (a) Should Ms. Petrie's employers have referred her?
   (b) What aspects of Ms. Petrie's conduct could have been given as a cause
       for concern as defined by the NMC?
   (c) What courses of action might the NMC have followed if she had been
       referred?

Following the investigation by the PCT, Ms. Petrie was reinstated to
her post.

Resources

NMC Code: https://www.nmc.org.uk/standards/code/read-the-code-
online/ (accessed 3/3/20)

NMC Fitness to Practice: https://www.nmc.org.uk/concerns-nurses-
midwives/dealing-concerns/what-is-fitness-to-practise/ (accessed 3/3/20)

Full article on this case. 'A Christian nurse suspended for offering to pray.'
Nursing Times 2.02.2009.

3.4   Patients and Carers   204

There is evidence that spiritual well-being is positively associated with health and   205
that providing spiritual support may enhance quality of life [22]. Patients/clients   206
have also been telling us for decades that the spiritual part of their life is important 207
to them, especially when facing life changing events such as illness [23–26]. Across   208
conditions and cultures, commonly reported needs include: to make sense of and to   209
adapt to their situation; to find hope and meaning in it and for the future; to stay   210
connected to self, others and the transcendent, rather than becoming isolated and   211
lonely; to be seen as a whole person, not just an illness/condition [27]. Carers report 212
similar needs, although few studies include them. So, patients/clients/carers have   213
called for what is most important to them to be acknowledged and addressed within   214
their care. In short, they want person-centred spiritual care; however, outside of the   215
specialist palliative care setting, this is seldom provided [28]. Many reasons have   216
been suggested for this gap in care provision including the busy clinical milieu of   217
frequently understaffed and financially constrained health services combined with a   218
focus on biomedical interventions in acute care [26].   219

Patients/carers see the nurse/midwife as one of the most appropriate healthcare   220
professionals to provide spiritual care [27]. This makes sense because patients are   221
likely to have the most contact with a nurse/midwife who frequently provides inti-   222
mate care, and therefore greater opportunity to establish trusting relationships out of 223
which deeper 'spiritual' conversations might emerge. It also makes sense because   224
the nurse/midwife is the advocate for the patient/client and signposts to other staff   225
and services including specialist spiritual support. Nurses/midwives see themselves   226
as having a key role in the provision of spiritual care (RCN survey, Table 3.2); it is   227
part of their remit set out by some regulatory and professional bodies, as outlined in   228
Sect. 3.3 above. The problem is that nurses/midwives report feeling least prepared   229
for this part of their role; a finding reported in large-scale surveys in the UK (RCN   230
Survey, Table 3.2), Australia [29] and New Zealand [30]. This feeling of inadequacy   231
may be another reason for patients' spiritual needs not being addressed. Box 3.3   232
invites you to consider whether a spiritual assessment is routinely included as part   233
of a patients' overall assessment where you work.   234

Box 3.3: Reflection Exercise 2

It is important to understand what spiritual care looks like for each patient.
Patients may not use the term 'spirituality'; hence, listening carefully to the
patient's vocabulary is important [12].

When did you last conduct a patient assessment? Was assessment of spiritual needs part of this? What questions are asked about spirituality on your
admission forms? Does this capture the real essence of spirituality as outlined
in the EPICC Standard? Might other wording be more appropriate? If spiritual assessment is not included in your overall assessment, why is that?

3.5 Nurses and Midwives

Nurses/midwives have been calling for over two decades for more education to better prepare them for spiritual care ([25, 31], RCN Survey Table 3.2). Although limited educational materials have been available for registered nurses/midwives (e.g. RCN Pocket Guide Table 3.2), the evidence on which they were based is scant, and they were not developed for students. There are a number of gaps in undergraduate spiritual care education:

1. Spiritual care teaching within undergraduate nursing/midwifery education programmes has been inconsistent, and in some places non-existent [31, 32].
2. It has been unclear what exactly should be included in curricula. Uncertainty about what spirituality is, what spiritual care looks like, what is reasonable to expect of nurses/midwives in provision of spiritual care and conflation of spirituality with religion have contributed to this lack of conceptual clarity. Media coverage of nurses being suspended by their regulatory body, as in the Caroline Petrie example above, for overstepping the mark has added to the confusion and fear of doing the wrong thing; better to do nothing than cause harm and risk losing one's job. Without conceptual clarity, it is difficult to decide on curriculum content.
3. The absence of evidence-based spiritual care competencies to provide guidance on the knowledge, skills and attitudes nurses/midwives need to demonstrate to be competent in spiritual care, separate from good nursing care.
4. Lack of clarity about what might help students to become competent in spiritual care, e.g. what factors contribute to development of competency? What helps learning? Box 3.4.

> **Box 3.4: Reflection for Educator**
> What is in your curriculum about spirituality and spiritual care? How is it taught? What works and what does not work? Are all four competencies in the EPICC Standard covered? How do you currently assess students' spiritual care competency in university and in clinical practice?

3.6 The Problem

Looking at the situation so far, we clearly have a problem that needs to be addressed which can be summarised as follows:

- Healthcare policy recognises the importance of people's spirituality for health and well-being.
- Patients/carers report unmet spiritual needs and would welcome spiritual care, especially from nurses. Spiritual well-being impacts positively on health and quality of life; spiritual support appears to enhance quality of life.

- Regulatory and professional bodies call for nurses/midwives to be competent in spiritual care.

But:

- Nurses and midwives do not feel competent in spiritual care and want more education.
- Spiritual care competencies are needed to assess nurses and midwives competence.
- Factors helping nurses/midwives to become competent in spiritual care need to be identified.

3.7 Responding to the Problem

3.7.1 International Research and Three Landmark European Studies (2010–2016)

Significant international work had already been undertaken on spiritual care education in nursing, summarised in three review papers. Ross [25] identified three studies conducted between 1983 and 2005, two from the UK and one from the Netherlands. In a repeat of [25] review, Cockell and McSherry [33] identified 10 further studies conducted between 2006 and 2010 in other European countries, North America and Brazil. In a review in 2015 specifically on pre-registration in nurse education and practice, Lewinson et al. [31] identified 28 studies conducted between 1992 and 2013 from Europe, North America, South Africa and the Far East. These studies highlighted that awareness of own spirituality may be a prerequisite for spiritual care and that educational courses may boost students/nurses confidence in and ability to assess for spiritual needs and to provide spiritual care. Some studies outlined the content and methods of course delivery. However, all of these studies were single centre and largely descriptive. There was a need to take stock of this evidence and to build upon it in a more organised and unified way.

To that end, the informal 'European Spirituality Research Network for Nursing and Midwifery' (a group of nurse/midwifery educators and researchers with an interest in spirituality) was established and conducted three robust international studies, summarised in McSherry et al. [34]. Two multi-centre studies (2010, 2011–2016) confirmed what the international literature had suggested that the personal spirituality of undergraduate nursing/midwifery students and how they perceived spirituality/spiritual care were key factors in the development of spiritual care competency. Students also identified what helped their learning about spiritual care; caring for patients was top of their list (see Box 3.5 for a student exemplar), followed by experience of personal life events and opportunity for discussion/teaching. A third study (2011–2015) developed a 54-item spiritual care competency framework for undergraduate nurses/midwives from the international literature, expert opinion and stakeholder engagement [36, 37].

Box 3.5: Student Exemplar

Caring for patients is important to students in learning about spiritual care. Here is an example from a student.

As part of spiritual care education, first year nursing students in two different nursing schools in Norway were given an assignment to use Stoll's assessment guide [35] to help them have a conversation about spiritual matters with a patient. The main themes in Stoll's assessment guide are: (1) sources of hope and strength, (2) relations between spiritual beliefs and health, (3) religious practices and concept of god or deity.

After the conversation, one of the students wrote this brief summary of the conversation and her own reflections.

I had a conversation with a former cancer patient, a woman aged 60–70 years. The first thing I explored was her (1) sources of hope and strength. It emerged that she had a lot of trust in other people. She visited her doctor about her illness, but family was also important for support. She said that when you get seriously ill, there is little you can do yourself. You have to trust the professionals around you and choose to think positively as far as possible.

She also told me that if she needed extra energy, hope or strength, it helped her stay in touch with nature. She needed to see the sea, smell the flowers, hear the sounds of birds chirping or go for a walk in the woods.

On the relationship between (2) spiritual beliefs and health, she said that she is generally an optimist, but that when she was diagnosed with cancer, she also saw the dark side of the life. 'Obviously you walk into the basement and think of death', she said. She had full confidence in the nurses and the doctors and felt well taken care of. She believed in medicine, skilled professionals and good information, and she felt safe. This provided her with meaning. Good information, explanations about how the medicines worked and what treatments would do to her were important.

Now she is a skinny older lady, and she believes that in the future she will age and her body will decay. But she said that 'it's okay when I know I'm being taken good care of'. Her greatest fear was not her cancer or old age, but rather being prone to injury or accident.

(3) She told me that she was raised in the Christian faith, but that she had no faith in Jesus or God today. She now considers herself a non-believer and is not a member of any religious denomination. She says she has no faith in the eternal reality. The only thing she believes in is the medicine, the doctors and the nurses.

She told me a story from when she was ill when her cousin came to visit with her family to pray for her. She felt this was intrusive, and she had to ask them to leave. She said she understood that it was important to them, but it was not what she needed.

Reflections on the conversation: When we were told about this assignment, I knew immediately who I wanted to talk to. I think it was a very interesting topic, and I thought it was great to have the opportunity to talk to someone about it. I thought that when you get sick and when the ground you are on disappears, then it would be good to have a faith in something bigger than yourself. The conversation with this cancer patient showed me that one does not necessarily have to be religious to believe in something. You can find meaning in the situation you are in.

This woman chose to believe in medicine and professionals, this gave her motivation and positive thoughts that 1 day she would be completely healthy. This is clearly something I will take with me into practice. It is permissible to believe in medicine, in God or in family or nature, and it is permissible to find something or someone to add extra trust to without necessarily having to be religious. This is something I think I would have liked to hear even if I was a non-religious patient who was experiencing illness and despair. Believing in something gives strength.

I also think that relatives, therapists and other people around the sick patient are important. You do not necessarily have to believe in the same thing to cooperate, but you can have a common goal and a shared hope that things will go well with help. If healthcare staff and family who are around the sick person only see the darkest in the dark when it is tough, then it might drain the patient of energy. It is important to support whatever the patient believes in, gives hope, mastery and faith.

At the same time, it is important not to let one's own beliefs override the patient's beliefs. As in the story of the cousin of this patient. The patient had an understanding of her cousin's faith, and that she wanted to pray for her, but it still felt intrusive and overwhelming. The patient had to ask her to leave. I think it is important that we have our own faith, and that the most important thing is that we support each other, even if we do not share the same belief. We have to respect what the patient believes, listen and understand. For me as a nursing student it may feel good if I can say that I believe in something bigger, but I must not let that interfere with patient care.

It was very interesting to talk to this lady about her illness. I dared to ask the difficult questions and it went well. Afterwards, I felt that the patient felt safe talking to me and that she felt heard and understood. I'm happy about that. The patient even called me up later in the evening to tell me a story she forgot to talk about earlier. The fact that she chose to call me even though we had ended the conversation told me something about how she experienced this conversation as important. And what's important to the patient is also important to us who work with them every day. All in all, I see this as a very educational and not least important topic. Everyone believes in something, but you may not be aware of your own beliefs before being asked. The woman I spoke with can tell that she believed in the knowledge and the people around her. Therefore, I think it is important that health professionals focus more on patients own faith. Maybe I can help the patient to find out what they believe in. Whether it is religious, science, love, the people around or other things. Finding something you can believe in provides security, hope, motivation and strength.

3.7.2   The EPICC Project (2016–2019)

This section cut down.

Erasmus K2+ funding enabled 31 nursing and midwifery educators from 21 European countries to work together to consider how the available research evidence might be pulled together to inform best practice in nurse/midwifery preregistration spiritual care education across Europe.

The four outputs from the EPICC Project, described in detail in Chap. 1, are starting to be recognised by those responsible for educating nurses and midwives. One example is Wales's commitment to embed the EPICC Spiritual Care Education Standard within all undergraduate nursing and midwifery programmes as outlined in Box 3.6.

The next step is to extend the work of EPICC beyond Europe to enhance best practice in spiritual care nurse/midwifery education globally. Steps in that direction are currently being taken through engagement with educators from China, Thailand and Brazil. We warmly invite others to join the EPICC Network to continue this important work.

> **Box 3.6: Exemplar of How EPICC Is Impacting on Undergraduate Nursing/Midwifery Education in One Country**
> At the EPICC Project Launch event On 1 July 2019 the Minister for Health & Social Services for Wales shared his vision for Wales to become the first compassionate country. The department commissioning pre-registration nursing/midwifery courses in Wales announced in July 2019 that all new nurse/midwifery courses in Wales will need to include the EPICC Standard. From 2020 all nursing/midwifery students in Wales will be assessed on the 4 EPICC spiritual care competencies in university and in clinical practice (https://heiw.nhs.wales/news/spiritual-care-to-become-part-of-welsh-nursing-curriculum/).

3.8   Summary of Main Points for Learning

This chapter has provided an overview of the different organisations and people that expect nurses and midwives to provide spiritual care as part of their wider holistic caring role. These include nurses and midwives themselves, the patients and carers they serve, nursing and midwifery professional/regulatory bodies, and healthcare policymakers. What exactly is expected of nurses and midwives, however, is not always clear, being clouded by differing interpretation in expectations and terminology. A number of exercises and case studies encourage the reader to reflect on some of these complexities and ambiguities for their own area of education and/or practice. However, what is clear is that nurses and midwives feel unprepared for spiritual care. This chapter outlines some resources

that have been produced from a decade of research to help to prepare student   333
nurses and midwives to become competent in spiritual care. Subsequent chap-   334
ters will focus on these resources in more detail.   335

References   336

1. World Health Organization. Handbook of resolutions and decisions 2 the determinants of   337
   health. Geneva: WHO; 1985. pp. 5–6.   338
2. World Health Organization. The spiritual dimension. Issue 9290211407; Chapter 4. 1991.   339
   http://www.worldebooklibrary.org/wplbn0000152153world-health-organization-publication-   340
   year-1991-issue-9290211407-chapter-26-by-world-healthorganization.aspx?   341
3. World Health Organization. WHOQOL and spirituality, religiousness and personal beliefs   342
   (SRPB). Social change and mental health cluster. Geneva: WHO; 1988. p. 4.   343
4. WHOQOL SRPB Group. A cross-cultural study of spirituality, religion, and personal beliefs   344
   as components of quality of life. Soc Sci Med. 2006;62:1486–97.   345
5. European Reference Networks. ERN assessment manual for applicants operational criteria for   346
   the assessment of healthcare providers. 2019. https://ec.europa.eu/health/sites/health/files/ern/   347
   docs/call2019_opcriteria_en.pdf.   348
6. Equality and Human Rights Commission. n.d.. https://www.equalityhumanrights.com/en/   349
   advice-and-guidance/religion-or-belief-discrimination. Accessed 30 Mar 2020.   350
7. Scottish Education Health Department. Guidelines on chaplaincy and spiritual care in the NHS   351
   in Scotland. 2002. https://www.sehd.scot.nhs.uk/mels/hdl2002_76.pdf.   352
8. Welsh Government. Health and care standards. Cardiff: Crown; 2015. http://www.wales.nhs.   353
   uk/sitesplus/documents/1064/24729_Health%20Standards%20Framework_2015_E1.pdf.   354
9. NHS England. NHS Chaplaincy Guidelines 2015 Promoting Excellence in Pastoral, Spiritual   355
   & Religious Care. 2015. https://www.england.nhs.uk/wp-content/uploads/2015/03/nhs-   356
   chaplaincy-guidelines-2015.pdf. Accessed 30 Mar 2020.   357
10. UK Board of Healthcare Chaplaincy. Standards for healthcare chaplaincy. 2009. https://www.   358
    ukbhc.org.uk/wp-content/uploads/2019/12/Encl-3-standards_for_healthcare_chapalincy_ser-   359
    vices_2009.pdf. Accessed 30 Mar 2020.   360
11. Nolan S, Saltmarsh P, Leget C. Spiritual care in palliative care: working towards an EAPC task   361
    force. Eur J Palliat Care. 2011;18(2):86–9.   362
12. Best M, Leget C, Goodhead A, Paal P. An EAPC white paper on multi-disciplinary education   363
    for spiritual care in palliative care. BMC Palliat Care. 2020;19(1):9. [PMID: 31941486].   364
13. Royal College of Psychiatrists. Recommendations for psychiatrists on spirituality and religion.   365
    Position Statement PS03/2013. London: RCP; 2013.   366
14. Nursing & Midwifery Council. The code. London: NMC; 2018a.   367
15. Nursing & Midwifery Council. Future nurse: standards of proficiency for registered nurses.   368
    London: NMC; 2018b.   369
16. Nursing & Midwifery Council. Standards of proficiency for midwives. London: NMC; 2019a.   370
17. Nursing & Midwifery Council. Standards for pre-registration midwifery programmes. London: 371
    NMC; 2019b.   372
18. Nursing & Midwifery Council. Standards framework for nursing and midwifery education.   373
    London: NMC; 2018c.   374
19. Ross L, McSherry W, Giske T, van Leeuwen R, Schep-Akkerman A, Koslander T, Hall J,   375
    Østergaard Steenfeldt V, Jarvis P. Nursing and midwifery students' perceptions of spiritual-   376
    ity, spiritual care, and spiritual care competency: a prospective, longitudinal, correlational   377
    European study. Nurse Educ Today. 2018;67:64–71.   378
20. McSherry W, Ross L. Spiritual shortfall? Nurs Stand. 2015a;29(35):22–3.   379
21. McSherry W, Ross L. Heed the evidence on place of spiritual needs in health care. Nurs Stand.   380
    2015b;29:38.   381

382 22. Balboni TA, Fitchett G, Handzo GF, et al. State of the science of spirituality and palliative
383   care research part II: screening, assessment and interventions. J Pain Symptom Manage.
384   2017;54:441–53.
385 23. Clark CC, Hunter J. Spirituality, spiritual wellbeing, and spiritual coping in advanced heart
386   failure. A review of the literature. J Holist Nurs. 2018;37(1):56–73.
387 24. Murray SA, Kendall M, Boyd K. Exploring the spiritual needs of people dying of lung cancer
388   or heart failure: a prospective qualitative interview study of patients and their carers. Palliat
389   Med. 2004;18(1):39–45.
390 25. Ross L. Spiritual care in nursing: an overview of the research to date. J Clin Nurs.
391   2006;15(7):852–62.
392 26. Ross L, Miles J. Spirituality in heart failure: a review of the literature from 2014 to 2019 to iden-
393   tify spiritual care needs and spiritual interventions. Curr Opin Palliat Care. 2020;14(1):9–18.
394   https://doi.org/10.1097/SPC.0000000000000475.
395 27. Selman LE, Brighton LJ, Sinclair S, Karvinen I, Egan R, Speck P, Powell RA, et al. Patients'
396   and caregivers' needs, experiences, preferences and research priorities in spiritual care: a focus
397   group study across nine countries. Palliat Med. 2018;32(1):216–30.
398 28. Royal College of Physicians (RCP). End of life care audit—dying in hospital: national report
399   for England 2016. London: RCP; 2016. https://www.rcplondon.ac.uk/projects/outputs/end-
400   life-care-audit-dying-hospital-national-report-england-2016. Accessed 18 Nov 2019.
401 29. Austin P, MacLeod R, Siddall P, McSherry W, Egan R. Spiritual care training is needed
402   for clinical and non-clinical staff to manage patients' spiritual needs. J Stud Spirituality.
403   2017;7(1):50–3. https://doi.org/10.1080/20440243.2017.1290031.
404 30. Egan R, Llewellyn R, Cox B, MacLeod R, McSherry W, Austin P. New Zealand nurses' per-
405   ceptions of spirituality and spiritual care: qualitative findings from a national survey. Religions.
406   2017;8(5):79. https://doi.org/10.3390/rel8050079.
407 31. Lewinson LP, McSherry W, Kevern P. Spirituality in pre-registration nurse education and prac-
408   tice: a review of the literature. Nurse Educ Today. 2015;35:806–14.
409 32. Ali G, Snowden M, Wattis J, Rogers M. Spirituality in nursing education: knowledge and
410   practice gaps. Int J Multidiscip Comparat Stud. 2018;5(1–3):27–49.
411 33. Cockell N, McSherry W. Spiritual care in nursing: an overview of published international
412   research. J Nurs Manag. 2012;20:958–69.
413 34. McSherry, W., Ross, L, Attard J, van Leeuwen R, Giske T, Kleiven T, Boughey A, the EPICC
414   Network. Preparing undergraduate nurses and midwives for spiritual care: some developments
415   in education over the last decade. J Stud Spirituality. 2020. https://doi.org/10.1080/2044024
416   3.2020.1726053.
417 35. Stoll RI. Guidelines for spiritual assessment. Am J Nurs. 1979;79:1574–77.
418 36. Attard J, Ross L, Weeks K. Design and development of a spiritual care competency frame-
419   work for pre-registration nurses and midwives: a modified Delphi study. Nurse Educ Pract.
420   2019a;39:96–104. https://doi.org/10.1016/j.nepr.2019.08.003.
421 37. Attard J, Ross L, Weeks K. Developing a spiritual care competency framework for pre-
422   registration nurses and midwives. Nurse Educ Pract. 2019b;40:102604. Advance online publi-
423   cation. https://doi.org/10.1016/j.nepr.2019.07.010.

Suggested Reading

425 European Association of Palliative Care. Spiritual care. https://www.eapcnet.eu/eapc-groups/
426   reference/spiritual-care
427 NHS Education for Scotland. Spiritual care. https://www.nes.scot.nhs.uk/education-and-training/
428   by-discipline/spiritual-care.aspx
429 Peng-Keller S, Neuhold D, editors. Charting spiritual care—the emerging role of chaplaincy
430   records in Global Healthcare. Cham: Springer Nature.
431 Timmins F, Caldeira S. Spirituality in healthcare: perspectives for innovative practice. Cham:
432   Springer Nature; 2019.

Chapter 4
Self-Care

Anthony Schwartz, Kath Baume, Austyn Snowden, Jyoti Patel, Nicky Genders, and Gulnar Ali

Learning Objectives

This chapter will enable you to:

1. Recognise emotional labour and reflect on how giving spiritual care has an impact on you as an individual.
2. Understand factors both internal and within the clinical environment that influence your self-care ability.
3. Develop and implement self-care strategies to ensure your on-going health and well-being.

A. Schwartz (✉)
Staffordshire University, Stoke-on-Trent, Staffordshire, UK
e-mail: Anthony.schwartz@staffs.ac.uk

K. Baume
Three Counties School of Nursing and Midwifery, University of Worcester, Worcester, UK
e-mail: k.baume@worc.ac.uk

A. Snowden
Mental Health, School of Health and Social Care, Edinburgh Napier University, Edinburgh, UK
e-mail: a.snowden@napier.ac.uk

J. Patel
SCPHN-OH Queen's Nurse, London, UK

N. Genders
University of South Wales, Newport, London, UK

G. Ali
New School of Psychotherapy and Counselling, London, UK

© Springer Nature Switzerland AG 2021
W. McSherry et al. (eds.), *Enhancing Nurses' and Midwives' Competence in Providing Spiritual Care*, https://doi.org/10.1007/978-3-030-65888-5_4

4.1   Introduction

A fundamental aim of nursing and midwifery is the protection and promotion of patients' mental, physical and spiritual well-being [1]. The nature of nursing and midwifery requires engagement in care of an emotional nature that is person centred and necessitates a sympathetic presence. To achieve a sympathetic presence requires you as a nurse or midwife to be present in the moment, talking and actively listening to understand a person's needs and wishes, respecting their privacy and dignity and providing support and reassurance, all of which are elements of spiritual care.

Much has been written about therapeutic relationships in nursing and midwifery, and one model that is repeatedly cited that underpins the development of trusting and collaborative relationship is Meutzel's model of therapeutic nurse–patient relationships [2]. The model describes three elements partnership, intimacy and reciprocity as overlapping circles identifying the point at which the circles coincide is where the therapeutic relationship arises.

Meutzel acknowledges the vulnerability of the person in the relationship and how the nurse through providing comfort can connect with the person creating a closeness of spirit through a sympathetic presence. Delivering spiritual care that treats a person as an individual, is compassionate and respects their values and feelings will ensure that any contact a nurse has with a patient is therapeutic [3]. Exploring the concept of reciprocity recognises that both the nurse and patient mutually benefit from the relationship, leading to the development of joint goals and improved patient outcomes [2]. It is recognised that helping people in need and providing compassionate care are sources of intrinsic motivation for becoming a nurse or midwife and whilst potentially emotionally demanding work, it can be challenging and have a positive effect on professional growth, motivation and well-being [4]. Developing self-awareness is essential to develop therapeutic relationships, and personal reflection can be a valuable tool in supporting your evolving practice and how you respond in different situations and recognise an individual's values, beliefs and attributes. Ali [5] emphasises that professional identity arises in conjunction with self-awareness of personal competencies and a commitment to practice standards.

4.1.1   Reflective Exercise

Reflective Exercise 1
Reflect on a situation where you provided intimate personal care and consider how the principles of Meutzel's therapeutic nurse–patient relationship was present in your practice?

Patients value compassionate care, and emotional work can result in compassionate satisfaction for nurses [6]. However, the emotional strain of caring, especially conducting difficult emotional encounters and meeting spiritual care needs, can result in nurses and midwives becoming emotionally depleted and can lead to compassion fatigue and burnout. Nurses and midwives are exposed to a variety of work stressors related to patient and family care giving which will vary according to the context of care. Nurses working in oncology will care for individuals living with the impact of long-term conditions and care for dying patients and their families who may wish to share their emotions, display grief and suffering with the emotional expectation that the nurse will support them towards a 'good death'. Similarly, nurses working in the emergency department caring for patients post trauma and supporting an individual and family's responses to life-changing injuries, resuscitation and near-death experiences require nurses to be emotionally responsive in a fast-paced unpredictable clinical environment. Each clinical specialty provides its own challenges for the nurse to balance the needs of the patient with the demands and interruptions of a busy work environment and staff shortages. Ultimately challenging environments can result in nursing and midwifery care falling short of the standards they hold, undermine their motivation and lead to burnout which is defined by Maslach and Jackson [7] as emotional exhaustion, depersonalisation and low levels of personal accomplishment.

A population survey of healthcare workers in Denmark found that midwives and homecare workers had high levels on both work- and client-related burnout yet those working in caseload midwifery had lower burnout scores and higher professional satisfaction [8]. Caseload midwifery is a model of care focusing on continuity, ensuring women receive all their care from one or only a few lead maternity carers or 'case loading midwives'.

Compassion fatigue occurs when nurses are no longer able to feel empathy towards people due to repeated exposure to others suffering [9] and has been described as emotional, physical and spiritual exhaustion from observing the problems and suffering of others [10]. Compassion fatigue can lead to physical symptoms such as decline in energy, headaches, anxiety and insomnia leading to absenteeism, low morale and poor job performance whilst burnout is associated with feelings of frustration, powerlessness and apathy due to the work environment, which can lead to compassion fatigue. Compassion fatigue can have a negative impact on person-centred care, patient satisfaction, patient safety, recruitment and retention and nurses' desire to leave the profession [9]. Consequently, nurses need to have increased awareness and recognition of compassion fatigue and burnout and develop coping strategies and interventions that promote rest, relaxation, exercise and social interaction to influence compassion satisfaction.

Emotional intelligence is the ability to understand one's own feelings, to empathise with the others' emotions, and to regulate an emotional response that is appropriate. The attribute of emotional intelligence is a significant factor in a nurses' understanding of emotional cues and body language, which is essential for effective person-centred care. Rouston [11] suggests nurses with high emotional intelligence have strong self-awareness and good interpersonal skills and are more empathetic, all attributes that are essential for developing therapeutic relationships. Emotional labour refers to the effort involved in managing feelings and expressions to fulfil the emotional requirements a role specifies, and the regulation of emotions displayed during interactions. The emotional nature of nursing and midwifery practice has been linked to emotional labour as nurses are expected to display empathetic outward emotions despite their inward feelings [12]. A conflict of emotions may arise, and nurses may disguise or suppress their emotions to align with the expectations of patients or colleagues and may lead to emotional dissonance. It is important to be aware of a range of human emotions that can be created due to uncertainty, such as those generated during wars, natural disasters and the Covid-19 pandemic. We can be guided through these uncertain times when it is difficult to verbalise the psychological impact of the intense feelings such as anticipatory grief and mourning [13].

4.1.2   Reflective Exercise

> **Reflective Exercise 2**
> *Reflect on a recent care episode where you provided person-centred care that was emotionally demanding.*
> - *How did you feel?*
> - *Was the experience rewarding and if so why?*
> - *How did you cope and process your emotional reactions to delivering the emotionally demanding care?*

4.2   Communication: Managing Difficult Situations

By analysing why people react to a stimulus in a particular way, it is possible to appreciate why some communication problems arise. Transactional analysis [14] provides a framework to explore this and is an important tool in the search for improved communications. In times of stress, our default behaviours that have been learnt are activated. What can be done to manage the complexity and effects of swirling demands and emotions—our own, the patients and their families. When handling difficult situations or interactions, we can only manage our own response to the behaviour we encounter. That means observing the behaviour, acknowledging it and dealing with it without reacting emotionally to it.

In challenging situations, is it important to accept that emotions exist, in themselves. How you or someone else feels about a situation is equally valid, yet can be entirely different from what others feel about the same situation. The emotions that exist can be generated from sources the patient or their families are not aware of. The question is, who is responsible for the feeling? The concern is if the nurse or midwife takes responsibility for the feelings expressed by families and patients (e.g. going into 'overdrive' trying to placate the other person, or spending a great deal of

time explaining and rationalising their positions). If the nurse and midwife can 113
accept it is okay for the family member or patient to have a feeling, they can stay in 114
the moment rather than stop them feeling what they are feeling. A lot of energy is 115
wasted on berating ourselves for having a feeling, rather than just accepting it.[1] 116

4.2.1 Reflective Exercise 117

Reflective Exercise 3
How do you respond when being challenged about something?
- *Is your response always appropriate?*
- *How do you respond to a critical friend?*
- *What are your default behaviours?*

Through examining the responses (e.g. are we focused on caring or critical 118
judgements, sharing information or expressing emotions), we can look for ways to 119
make changes. This is a way of raising awareness of the patterns that impact and 120
affect performance, and well-being. 121

On a daily basis, nurses and midwives are challenged by poor staffing levels, 122
high workload environments and the expectation to deliver care to those who may 123
be in emotional turmoil and pain which creates the potential for intense and stressful 124
experiences. There is a need to find a balance between work and private life and 125
encourage gathering support from experienced colleagues in order to achieve this. 126
Developing compassion for oneself may promote self-care and reduce self-criticism, 127
compassion fatigue and burnout. Nurses and midwives need to be kind to themselves. 128

Neff [15] conceptualised self-compassion as self-kindness, a sense of humanity 129
and mindfulness which involves 'being touched by and open to one's own suffering, 130
not avoiding or disconnecting from it, generating the desire to alleviate one's suffer- 131
ing and to heal oneself with kindness'. 132

4.3 Compassionate Self-Care and Resilience 133

The ability to reduce the risk of burnout and compassion fatigue has been associated 134
with an individual's emotional resilience. Within the clinical environment, the need 135
for emotional support and the opportunity to emotionally vent are key strategies to 136
support nurses to cope with the emotional demands of caring [16]. Furthermore, 137

---

[1] Thanks to Eamonn Dennis MD of The Conflict Training Company in the UK for his contribution on managing emotions in challenging situations.

138   when engaging in care that is emotionally draining, nurses need to draw on personal
139   resources and self-care ability to recognise emotional and physical fatigue in them-
140   selves and take proactive steps to replenish their emotions to avoid compassion
141   fatigue. One such resource maybe your personal spiritual well-being which Arnetz
142   et al. [17] identified as a mechanism for coping with stress and life difficulties, and
143   as a way of reducing emotional exhaustion and depersonalisation. In addition, it
144   may be helpful to consider other job resources such as coaching, performance feed-
145   back and social support and the impact that these factors may have on resilience.

146   ## 4.3.1   Reflective Exercise

Reflective Exercise 4
Consider your current work environment.
- *What factors exist that could lead to compassion fatigue?*
- *What self-care and work-based resources can you identify that will
  support your compassion satisfaction?*

147   The issue of self-compassion and self-care is explored by the Sophie Model [5]
148   which is a tool for reflexivity and self-inquiry and can be seen as framework for
149   self-care.

150   ## 4.4   Where Are You in This? Self-Care and Spirituality

151   Nursing and midwifery involve working in partnership with people, and we have
152   seen that this involves emotional labour; *being there* with patients, listening with an
153   empathic, non-judgmental attitude. We have discussed the importance of compas-
154   sion, emotional intelligence and resilience and their counterparts, burnout and com-
155   passion fatigue. These essentially spiritual elements of nursing will become
156   increasingly important as nursing continues to move away from routine, task-based
157   work towards creative asset-based solutions. But there is no doubt that this is an
158   essentially *spiritual* agenda. Compassion is emotional labour involving the active
159   use of self to help people in spiritual distress. This means we need to recognise
160   spiritual distress in others. It also means we need to look after our own spiritual
161   needs; to avoid compassion fatigue or burnout. So, how do we recognise spiritual
162   distress in others? Just as importantly, how would you know you were in spiritual
163   distress?

One way of recognising spiritual distress is therefore through *assessment*, only   164
in this case, instead of assessing someone else, the subject of the assessment is   165
going to be you.   166

4.4.1 How to Conduct a Spiritual Assessment on Yourself   167

There are many ways of conducting spiritual assessments, and these are discussed   168
widely throughout the book. Here we focus on a very short, five-item measure origi-   169
nally designed to help chaplains understand when their interventions have been suc-   170
cessful, the Scottish PROM [18]. Chaplains are specialists in delivering spiritual   171
care so by understanding how and when you would refer someone to specialist spiri-   172
tual care, you also understand criteria for assessing your own spiritual well-being.   173

Often we interpret or diagnose as part of our job, often with the best intentions,   174
but in doing so we can lose the essence of what people are trying to tell us. By con-   175
trast, the PROM helped chaplains discuss individual cases with colleagues when   176
reflecting on practice by reflecting on what patients actually say.   177

4.4.2 Reflective Exercise   178

Reflective Exercise 5
*Think of a time when you felt you 'connected' to a patient when you were
with them.*
- *When communicating and feeding back the conversation with the
  patients at a hand-over did you use the same language as patients had?*
- *What did you notice about your language and the interaction when it
  went well?*
- *Can you think of a previous occasion where you felt you struggled to
  engage with the patient, what happened?*
- *What do you think made a difference and enabled you to connect
  with the patient?*

The Scottish PROM consists of five questions (Box 4.1). First, you reflect on the   179
previous 2 weeks and then record how often you have felt: honest, anxious, positive, in   180
control and peaceful. These questions are rated on a 5-point scale from 'none of the   181
time' through to 'all of the time'. Each of the five item responses are then scored from   182
0 to 4, with 'anxiety' scored the other way around (4 to 0), because less anxiety is better   183
in this case. The total of all five items is calculated by adding the scores together.   184

Box 4.1: Scottish PROM©

In the last 2 weeks, I have felt...	None of the time	Rarely	Some of the time	Often	All the time	
I could be honest with myself about how I was really feeling	○	○	○	○	○	t1.1 t1.2 t1.3 t1.4
Anxious	○	○	○	○	○	t1.5
I had a positive outlook on my situation	○	○	○	○	○	t1.6 t1.7
In control of my life	○	○	○	○	○	t1.8
A sense of peace	○	○	○	○	○	t1.9
Finally, please add any further comments you wish to make:						t1.10

Scores range from 0 to 20, and the average score from the thousands of people who have completed it so far is close to 12. In general, anything under 10 therefore usually appears to indicate a degree of spiritual distress [19]. Of course, as with any psychometric measure, people vary in their responses and interpretation of the items, so scores need to be interpreted with caution. As part of a wider assessment, the PROM has proved very helpful in detecting spiritual distress and identifying people for whom a chaplaincy referral may be beneficial. If you score considerably less than 10, you may want to consider getting an appointment with the local chaplain. They are there to help you and all the staff, so do talk to them.

4.4.3   Reflective Exercise

Reflective Exercise 6
Spend 5 minutes completing the PROM (Box 4.1).
- *Did your result surprise you?*
- *Do you think you could use this to identify your spiritual distress?*

Recognising that the spiritual dimension in care when looking after other people and ourselves is fundamental. Consider your own well-being: What is important to you right now, in terms of looking after yourself? What helps you get up in the morning and keeps you mentally, emotionally, physically and spiritually healthy? While spiritual care has been widely researched, some nurses can find it challenging to implement in their everyday practice [3]. How do you manage to stay close to the patient, reflect empathy and practice 'active listening'? What do you need for yourself in order to be able to do this? What gets in the way? How can you promote a sense of calm interest when in an emotionally charged and busy situation?

Spiritual care has been associated with the words 'love' and 'kindness'. If patients [204] with cancer, their families and friends think this, and nurses caring for the patients [205] are considered to give this, what do you need so that you too can be 'loving' and [206] 'kind'? [3]. If you harness these elements within yourself, you can be fully authentic, and others will sense this and respond accordingly. Authenticity is reflected [208] through congruence, unconditional compassion and empathy for others. This is supported by the work of Carl Rogers and Martinsen [20] who assert that it requires [210] authenticity to develop meaningful and empathetic relationship with others. If you [211] are comfortable within yourself, you are likely to be available to others. Empathic [212] responding is made possible by a special group of nerve cells called mirror neurons [213] at various places in the brain [21]. This ability comes from within us. It allows us to [214] understand another person's feelings and thoughts or situation as they experience it. [215]

4.5 You Make the Difference: The Nurse as a Healthy Resource [216] [217]

The work you do is valuable and impacts on those you treat, and the wider community. It is something you have devoted yourself to, given time and energy to, and [219] in which you are clearly invested. No doubt you also gain a sense of personal and [220] job satisfaction from what you do. It takes skill, energy, emotional effort and time to [221] work effectively with people, and you do it. What do you need to be able to keep on [222] doing it and do you make space and time for that? [223]

Bettison [22] recognises that whilst midwives provide emotional 'holding' in [224] their working roles, they often do not get hold and contain themselves. People working in healthcare assist people, and generally put their own needs to the side, making [226] sure that others are looked after. [227]

Whilst engaging and meeting the needs of others is part of the vocation of nursing, much of this is not a conscious decision, but something you do from within. The [229] emphasis is often on the safety of those in our care; however, there needs to be [230] recognition of the carers' well-being in this safety critical profession [23]. If a nurse [231] is experiencing ill health, this may compromise their capacity to be appropriately [232] caring and effective. In the UK, there is legislation and regulation for employers [233] about health and safety in the workplace (e.g. Management of Health and Safety at [234] Work Regulations 1999). The Health and Safety Executive (HSE) advises employers to develop work cultures where 'good health is good business', as health/wellbeing, reduces sickness absence, improves productivity and helps to retain staff at [237] work. All this makes an organisation more effective. [238]

In March [24], The Royal College of Nursing (RCN) launched the '3Rs' campaign to encourage nurses to 'rest, refresh and rehydrate' during shifts in recognition that nursing workforce shortages were resulting in nursing staff missing their [241] breaks. Currently, staff/personnel shortages and increasing workloads create a tension or dissonance at the 'frontline' of nursing, self-care and taking a break versus [243] implementing required patient/client care, which is further supported by the WHO [244] [25] Covid-19 healthcare guidelines. Nurses and midwives need to assert [245]

246   themselves to take self-care actions at work, recognising that if other staff/personnel
247   are not taking breaks, then it can be much harder to consider their own needs and
248   say 'I need to step away to eat, or take a rest or get a drink'.

249   ## 4.5.1   Reflective Exercise

> **Reflective Exercise 7**
> *Take a look at RCN 3Rs campaign https://www.rcn.org.uk/magazines/acti-*
> *vate/2018/march/rest-rehydrate-refuel*
> *   Consider your last clinical placement: was there a culture that enabled*
> *the 3 R's?*
> - *If yes how was this embedded into the clinical day?*
> - *If this did not occur what were the barriers and how did you feel?*
> - *Moving forward into your next placement what strategies could you*
>   *adopt to ensure you had a rest break, drinks, and time to eat?*

250   So because of increasing work pressures, it is more important than ever for
251   nurses and midwives to be aware of and routinely implement their own spiritual
252   self-care plan particularly outside of work. There is a need to develop a clear delin-
253   eation between work and personal life, for example being a clear on our boundaries.
254   The delineation gives work-free time during which nurses and midwives can focus
255   on their own health/well-being needs as much as possible which in turn helps them
256   to sustain their own practice and be fit for work.
257   One practical way to do this is to be aware of routines which overtly and clearly
258   indicate that 'work is complete'. For example, at end of a shift, nurses and midwives
259   undertake actions which denote 'work is complete' and personal time begins. A
260   clear routine undertaken mindfully (keeping self-care in mind) can create a bound-
261   ary between work and non-work time.
262   The following is a suggested routine (adapted from [26]) as a way of a nurse or
263   midwife completing the shift and moving into their own life:

> **Reflective Exercise 8**
> *Write down what needs to be remembered and/or complete/update contempo-*
> *raneous clinical notes, then complete verbal handover of patient care and*
> *give good-byes. These actions formally indicate the end of professional*
> *responsibilities.*
> - *Wash hands (from elbow to fingertips) and change clothing before*
>   *leaving the workplace to physically signal the end of a shift (it is also*
>   *good infection control).*

- *Then mindfully head away from work, whilst connecting with your body on the way—notice how your body feels (tired, light, relief to be sitting down whilst travelling, etc.). Ideally head towards a pre-planned supportive activity of connection e.g. exercise, being in nature, seeing family/friends, eating a favourite meal.*
- *Include time for rest/sleep before the next shift.*

Using the above example, plan your own 'end of work' and beginning of work routines.

It is recognised that self-care is necessary and legitimate. Likis [27] in her editorial challenges' midwives to 'make themselves a priority with a focus on the self-care, self-love, and realistic expectations that we teach our patients about daily' (p. 9).

As an individual perhaps you can do things on your own, but increasingly there are workplace stress-management and other supports available (e.g. well-being policies, health-related advice and counselling services). Thinking about self-care, there are some activities and strategies you can do as a preventative approach (building in healthy activities such as walking, reading, etc.) others to help restore your well-being (rest, refuel and rehydrate) and finally ones that can be used as rehabilitation if you have encountered a crisis (counselling, therapy and developing long-term self-care strategies). Once you are on track with your own well-being and self-care plan, it is important to find ways of maintaining that energy and reminding yourself of the skills you have learnt.

4.5.2 Reflective Exercise

Reflective Exercise 9

Consider the previous time out activities and the impact on your personal emotional well-being.

- *Reflect on where you are along the cycle of change regarding self-care.*
- *Are you aware of a 'cue to action' that has been triggered in practice?*
- *What feelings has this created in you?*
- *How can you develop self-care strategies to manage these feelings?*
- *What form can these approaches take that fit with you?*
- *If you have implemented new ways of being and a 'blip' occurs, can you be kind to yourself and 'regroup' so that you can carry on?*
- *How will you ensure these self-care strategies become part of your routine moving forward?*

278   ## 4.6   Strategies for Self-Care: Self-Discovery, Self-Reflection
279   and Self-Care

280   As nurses our socilisation and education focuses on the care we provide towards
281   others. This includes understanding the impact of empathy, kindness and compas-
282   sion on the well-being of others. Self-care is at the heart of enabling others through
283   ensuring we have the capacity to offer what our patients need at times when we feel
284   challenged. Robinson [28] cautions that 'the nurse who avoids self-reflection will
285   eventually tire of agitation, burn-out, or be undone by her tears when she looks in
286   the mirror. It's never too late to move towards consciousness' (p. 184).

287   ### 4.6.1   Exploration of Self

288   As part of a reflexive process, the exploration of who we are, is important, in the
289   context of our working environment but also beyond. Am I a nurse for my working
290   day or is this who I am as a person 24 h a day and what does this mean? Is being a
291   nurse a role, a job or who you are as a person? Often when we explore the self, we
292   ignore the self in specific contexts. For example, I may describe myself in relation
293   to my roles but also my characteristics. I may describe myself as strong but is this
294   in all contexts, in every situation or at all times? Probably not is the answer to that.
295   However, recognising that is important, knowing when I might not be 'strong' but
296   also understanding what that means to me when I describe myself as such is part of
297   the exploration of self. Nurses and midwives are caring? patient? resilient? strong?
298   But when we are faced with these views and we feel we do not hold these character-
299   istics all of the time, how does that shape how we see ourselves? A realistic view of
300   self therefore helps us to hold more realistic expectations of ourselves too.

301   ### 4.6.2   Reflection on Self and Health: How Am I Doing?

302   We often notice when our physical health causes us a concern but do we pay atten-
303   tion to our mental, emotional and spiritual health? What does good health look like
304   to you in this context? How do you feel at the end of a 12-h shift at work? How do
305   you feel on your days away from work? Understanding yourself and who you are in
306   different contexts will help you to identify our own concerns about potential changes
307   in our physical, psychological and mental health.

308   ### 4.6.3   Actions: Self-Care Techniques

309   Part of the process of self-care is to identify strategies that can help maintain or
310   enhance well-being. These are individual to you and should come about after
311   reflection and self-exploration. Examples of self-care techniques include time to

be alone, walking in nature, exercise routines, swimming, yoga, meditation, 312
massage or reading; in addition to the physical activity, we can also include 313
activities like talking with friends, going to church or positive thinking. Peer 314
group discussions, personal supervision, coaching and counselling are other 315
forms of self-care; particularly the ability to be able to 'let go' of mental and 316
emotional baggage (for more information, explore Acceptance and Commitment 317
Therapy approaches, [29]). 318

4.6.4 Mindfulness 319

Mindfulness can be described as paying particular attention in a particular 320
manner, to a particular moment using a non-judgemental accepting approach 321
[30] in [31]. As intervention, mindfulness can be used to support mental well- 322
being; however, it is a 'practice' requiring 'practice'. In the context of self-care 323
in the caring professions, mindfulness can offer the opportunity to be 'present' 324
and non-judgemental of a given situation. Executive coaching using mindful- 325
ness is one way of gaining insight and changing behaviour to enhance well- 326
being [32]. 327

4.6.5 Music and Creative Arts Expression 328

Applications of creative arts' strategies (music, singing, literature, writing and art) 329
are seen to be ameliorative and can enhance well-being. Gillam [33] shows that 330
creativity and well-being are fundamental to reducing occupational stress and pro- 331
moting professional satisfaction, and reduces levels of stress, and there has been 332
beneficial use of music and singing with different patient groups. One wellness 333
trend for staff at risk of being overwhelmed by stress is the teaching of musical 334
instruments or singing at work (www.musicinoffices.com). Anecdotally, we all 335
know how music affects our own mood and so it too, is something we can recom- 336
mend as part of the range of self-care strategies. 337

4.6.6 Meditation 338

A century-old technique meditation has been used both within and outside of 339
religious practices. 'Meditation is the ability to quieten the mind and focus 340
thoughts inwards through relaxed concentration upon a chosen stimulus' ([34], 341
p. 79). Often health benefits described arise from the deep relaxation that those 342
who practice meditation can be achieved. As part of meditative practice visuali- 343
sation may be used which can deepen relaxation or distract from negative 344
thoughts. 345

4.6.7 Yoga

Yoga has existed as a practice for centuries with growing popularity in the West as the link between mind and body became more widely accepted [34]. Yoga practice is often separated into 'schools' or forms which have their own set of postures and mantras, and may link in with meditations. In the West, yoga has often been seen as a form of exercise; however, evidence suggests that breathing, meditation and visualisation used in some forms of yoga can enhance well-being and can particularly be used as a self-care strategy for nurses and midwives.

4.6.8 Exercise

It has been consistently demonstrated that physical exercise has considerable physical, psychological, and social benefits, and the World Health Organisation (WHO) has Global Recommendations on Physical Activity for Health [35]. Whilst many nursing, midwifery and medical students do not meet physical activity guidelines, professionals are often regarded as 'role models' for health. We may usefully consider how our own behaviours and physical activity habits may influence those whom we treat and quality of the service we provide.

At least a half an hours' exercise daily is encouraged. Aside from increasing overall health and well-being, improving self-esteem and a sense of personal accomplishment, exercise has direct stress-relieving advantages. It has physiological and neurochemical benefits, e.g. releasing endorphins. Aerobic exercise improves the ability to sleep, which is a cornerstone of health and well-being, is good for the heart and helps us to feel energised. Formal gym work-outs and physical activity programmes can be helpful to develop overall fitness and are to be encouraged. What we often forget is how to include activity and physical exertion in our everyday lives. It is natural, we can include it in our routines, and the old adage runs true: A little is better than none! Although it may be a challenge to slot exercise into your routine in the beginning, remember that a good habit takes around 3–6 weeks to become established and embedded. If you begin by not being in shape, once you begin to tolerate exercise, you may find you then start to enjoy it, and ultimately it becomes something you do not want to be without. Most of all, the neurotransmitters released through exercise help give a 'feel-good factor'.

4.6.9 Practical Time Out Opportunity

The reason you would take a time out is:

• If you are starting to notice any signs of 'burnout' or 'mental fatigue', this is when you are aware that you are not fully focused on the task in hand or functioning to your full potential.

- Being able to take you away from your 'clinical brain' and allowing yourself to switch off from the clinical environment enabling self-care mode.
- Doing this 'time out' regime, facilitates a clear mind which enables you to re-evaluate and restructure priorities and workloads within the clinical area, away from the immediate pressures that could influence your decision-making process.

Take time out to do some basic leg, back and shoulder stretches and exercises. All these can be done in the clinical environment, e.g. staff room or hand over area. If the ward/department has a changing room facility, then that is ideal.

Let us start with the legs: they potentially are tired and aching, and you may have sore feet (being on them for the best part of the morning shift, and still aching from the long day's overtime yesterday). Possibly your mind is not 110% concentrating, and you have got the 14.00-h drug round to do.

This would be the perfect opportunity to have a 'self-care time out' (see Box 4.2). A drink of water with 5 min of stretching and exercise. This will enable the focus back on the task, as it will relieve or at least help reduce the effect of the distraction (aching legs, back, etc.) from the task in hand, enabling a new fresh focus on the drug round, thus reducing the risk of a 'near miss' or a drug error to a patient from the administration point.

4.6.10   Five-Minute Self-Care Time out Break

Box 4.2: Factors you Will Need to Consider Facilitating your 5-Minute 'Physical and Mental Self-Care' Time Out [36]
- Use exercises that will give you the most beneficial outcome, e.g. calf raises to reduce venous pooling.
- Situational awareness.
- Stretches and exercises.
- Tailor your exercises to the environment you are in.
- Remember rehydration.
- Sustain healthy balanced food intake throughout the shift.
- Ensure you create 5 min 'self-care time out' when you feel the effects of 'burnout' or 'mental fatigue'.
- Enable yourself to be an advocate for best safe practice within your clinical area.

A final part of the process of self-care should include sustainable strategies. Maintaining well-being in the nursing and midwifery context is an ongoing process, requiring review of the techniques and strategies that work (or do not work) for you, and a focus on their sustainability. Choosing a strategy that is right for you (and you know you can sustain) can build your self-care toolkit. Bloom's 'Your Spiritual

407   Health Programme' (YSHP) helps an individual identify actions and gently reflect-
408   ing on areas of spiritual self-care such as being in nature, exercising, being with
409   family/friends, etc. (YSHP https://yourspiritualhealth.org/).

410   ## 4.7   Cue to Action

411   One of the most helpful applied psychology models when considering making
412   changes is the Transtheoretical Model of Change described first by Prochaska and
413   DiClemente [37] which suggests movement through predictable well-defined stages
414   (see Box 4.3), recognising there will be 'blips' or relapses along the way. The model
415   is best depicted by an upward spiral representing movement through the consecu-
416   tive stages of change, as opposed to assuming a linear progression from start to
417   finish.

Box 4.3: Transtheoretical Model of Change [37]

Pre-Contemplation	No real awareness of the need to change until a **Cue to Action** arises Something happens either externally or internally that triggers you to recognise the need to change	Self-care not on your agenda or important to you until A crisis occurs of you are being challenged by situation or colleague and you feel less resilient	t2.1 t2.2 t2.3 t2.4 t2.5 t2.6 t2.7
Contemplation	Recognise and think about change	Aware of events and signs of stress, anxiety, depression or burnout or physical symptoms [38]	t2.8 t2.9 t2.10
Determination/planning	Laying the foundations for change, planning what it is needed	Begin to plan or prepare for self-care and want to make changes. This is about laying the foundations for change What it is that is needed or what you need to do next. When, how and where, and who may be involved	t2.11 t2.12 t2.13 t2.14 t2.15 t2.16 t2.17
Action	Doing what you have committed to	Being proactive, talking to someone, re-engaging in things that are good for you like walking, singing, taking physical exercise, enjoying music, taking part in community, social or spiritually uplifting activities	t2.18 t2.19 t2.20 t2.21 t2.22 t2.23
Maintenance	Keep going with the new behaviours / activities	Continue with routines and healthy habits. Doing what you find supports your self-care and well-being (e.g. including fitness activities, sustaining personal boundaries, social activity, finding solitude in nature, etc.)	t2.24 t2.25 t2.26 t2.27 t2.28 t2.29

Through adopting self-care strategies, you can actively start to monitor their impact on yourself (e.g. feeling less gloomy, having regained a sense of inspiration, mentally feeling more in control). One thing we may all recognise is that pressures in life and work are dictating the pace, and we do not easily allow ourselves time out and time for ourselves (even to discover our needs, as we usually just plough on, and this can lead to avoidance activities and a lead to a crisis).

A word of caution: from time to time despite our best actions and intentions, we can get stuck, or have a 'blip' or relapse. This may feel like we are back where we started. What is encouraging about this model is that we can never get back to the pre-contemplation stage but will need to think our self-care changes along the continuum between the contemplation, planning/determination, action and maintenance stages. We may even recognise that our actions were good, but perhaps the timing was not ideal. For instance if we start a new lifestyle activity (e.g. when we get back to running which we used to find a good way of 'switching off'), the season we begin to do this may make it harder or easier to follow through. It is also important to recognise that "blips" may occur due to external factors beyond your control (e.g. winter pressures on staff in hospital and sickness in teams may impede opportunities for self-care). We may thereby create a 'virtuous cycle' that helps you and at the same time enables virtuous nursing practice [1].

4.8 Summary

The nature of nursing and midwifery requires engagement in therapeutic relationships of an emotional nature and necessitates a sympathetic presence. The emotional strain of caring, difficult emotional encounters and meeting spiritual care needs, can result in nurses and midwives becoming emotionally depleted and can lead to compassion fatigue and burnout. In this chapter, we have recognised the importance of self-care as essential to working as a nurse or midwife. Finding the resources and strategies which are right for you to enhance your resilience is key to maintaining personal and professional well-being. If we do not recognise and take action to promote care of oneself, we will never be able to meet the spiritual needs of people in our care.

References

1. Jubilee Centre for Character and Virtues. Virtuous practice in nursing. 2017. http://www.jubileecentre.ac.uk/1588/projects/current-projects/virtuous-practice-in-nursing. Accessed 20 Dec 2019.
2. Richardson C, Percy M, Hughes J. Nursing therapeutics: teaching student nurses care, compassion and empathy. Nurse Educ Today. 2015; https://doi.org/10.1016/j.nedt.2015.01.01.
3. Clarke J, Baume K. Embedding spiritual care into everyday nursing practice. Nurs Stand. 2019. https://doi.org/10.7748/ns.2019.e11354.

456   4. Donoso LM, Demerouti E, Hernández EG, Moreno-Jiménez B, Cobo IC. Positive benefits of
457   caring on nurses' motivation and well-being: a diary study about the role of emotional regula-
458   tion abilities at work. Int J Nurs Stud. 2015;52:804–16.
459   5. Ali G. Multiple case studies exploring integration of spirituality in Undergraduate Nursing
460   Education in England. Doctoral thesis, University of Huddersfield; 2017. http://eprints.hud.
461   ac.uk/id/eprint/34129/.
462   6. Hooper C, Craig J, Janvrin DR, et al. Compassion satisfaction, burnout, and compassion
463   fatigue among emergency nurses compared with nurses in other selected inpatient specialties.
464   J Emerg Nurs. 2010;36(5):420–7.
465   7. Maslach C, Jackson S. The measurement of experienced burnout. J Organ Behav.
466   1981;2:99–113. https://doi.org/10.1002/job.4030020205.
467   8. Jepsen I, Juul S, Foureur M, Sørensen E, Nøhr E. Is caseload midwifery a healthy work-form?
468   A survey of burnout among midwives in Denmark. Sex Reprod Healthc. 2016;11:102–6.
469   9. Peters E. Compassion fatigue in nursing: a concept analysis. Nurs Forum. 2018; https://doi.
470   org/10.1111/nuf.12274.
471   10. Sabo B. Reflecting on the concept of compassion fatigue. Online J Issues Nurs. 2011;16(1):1–22.
472   https://doi.org/10.3912/OJIN.Vol16No01Man01.
473   11. Rouston J. Emotional intelligence: an essential skill for nurses. 2010. https://www.healthecar-
474   eers.com/article/career/emotional-intelligence-an-essential-skill-for-nurses.
475   12. Elliott C. Emotional labour: learning from the past, understanding the present. Br J Nurs.
476   2017;26(19):1070–7. https://doi.org/10.12968/bjon.2017.26.19.1070.
477   13. Bertinato S. That discomfort you are feeling. Harvard Bus Rev. 2020. https://hbr.org/2020/03/
478   that-discomfort-youre-feeling-is-grief.
479   14. Berne E. Games people play: the psychology of human relationships. New York: Grove
480   Press; 1964.
481   15. Neff KD. The development and validation of a scale to measure self-compassion. Self Identity.
482   2003;2:223–50. https://doi.org/10.1080/15298860309027.
483   16. Kinman G, Leggetter S. Emotional labour and wellbeing: what protects nurses? Healthcare.
484   2016;4:89. https://doi.org/10.7748/ns.2019.e11354.
485   17. Arnetz B, Ventimiglia M, Beech P, Demarinis V, Lökk J, Arnetz J. Spiritual values and prac-
486   tices in the workplace and employee stress and mental well-being. J Manage Spiritual Religion.
487   2013;10:271–81. https://doi.org/10.1080/14766086.2013.801027.
488   18. Lobb EA, Schmidt S, Jerzmanowska N, Swing AM, Thristiawati S. Patient reported outcomes
489   of pastoral care in a hospital setting patient reported outcomes of pastoral care in a hospi-
490   tal setting. J Health Care Chaplain. 2018;25:131–46. https://doi.org/10.1080/08854726.201
491   8.1490059.
492   19. Snowden A, Telfer I. Patient reported outcome measures of spiritual care as delivered by
493   chaplains. J Health Care Chaplain. 2017;23(4):131–55. https://doi.org/10.1080/08854726.201
494   7.1279935.
495   20. Brown B. Daring greatly—how the courage to be vulnerable transforms the way be live, love,
496   parent and Lead. New York: Gotham; 2012.
497   21. Keysers C. The empathic brain. Chicago: University of Chicago Press; 2011.
498   22. Bettison H. Caring for the carer, healing the healer: the importance of self care and support for
499   midwives. Women Birth. 2019;32(sup 1):S45. Accessed 3 Mar 2020. https://doi.org/10.1016/j.
500   wombi.2019.07.286.
501   23. Leary A. Safety and service. Reframing the purpose of nursing to decision makers.
502   Editorial. 2016. https://openresearch.lsbu.ac.uk/download/d4dd89a21ff1f1b5f3bcac9004b
503   f3f21872054d5e3987b854e79c7f247a1f703/115514/JCNEditorialMay2017.pdf. Orcid
504   ID: 0000-0001-7846-5658. https://www.wcmt.org.uk/sites/default/files/report-documents/
505   Leary%20A%20Report%202016%20Final.pdf
506   24. Royal College of Nursing. Rest, rehydrate and refuel. 2018. https://www.rcn.org.uk/
507   news-and-events/news/new-campaign-urges-nursing-staff-to-take-rest-breaks.

25. World Health Organisation. Mental health and psychosocial considerations during the COVID-19outbreak. 2020. https://www.who.int/docs/default-source/coronaviruse/mental-health-considerations.pdf.

26. Whittle A-M. Alexander Filmer-Lorch et al. (chapter 29) the inner power of stillness: a practical guide for therapists and practitioners. London: Handspring; 2016.

27. Likis FE. Self-care: taking care of ourselves to optimize the care we provide. J Midwifery Womens Health. 2016;61(1):9–10.

28. Robinson E. The soul of the nurse. Santa Barbara, CA: Spann Robinson; 2013.

29. Hayes SC, Strosahl KD, Wilson KG. Acceptance and commitment therapy: the process and practice of mindful change. 2nd ed. New York: The Guilford Press; 2012.

30. Kabat-Zinn J. Coming to our senses: Healing ourselves and the world through mindfulness. London: Hachette; 2005.

31. Comperat JM, Genders N. Resource buddy: developing an online resource to support mindfulness-based interventions for people with learning disabilities. Learn Disabil Pract. 2019;22(5)

32. Schwartz AL. Mindfulness in applied psychology; building resilience in coaching. Coach Psychol. 2018;14(2):98–104.

33. Gillam T. Enhancing public mental health and wellbeing through creative arts participation. J Public Ment Health. 2018;17(4):148–56. https://doi.org/10.1108/jpmh-09-2018-0065.

34. Genders N. Fundamental aspects of complementary therapies for health care professionals. London: Quay Books; 2006.

35. World Health Organization. Global recommendations on physical activity for health. Geneva, Switzerland: World Health Organization; 2010.

36. Palmer N. Personal communication—health and wellbeing coaching: how to include exercise for self-care in nurses and midwives. 2020.

37. Prochaska JO, DiClemente CC. Trans-theoretical therapy: towards a more integrative model of change. Psychother Theor Res Pract. 1982;19:276–88.

38. Chambers et al. Beating stress in the NHS. Radcliffe Medical Press, Oxford. 2003.

39. Adimando A. Preventing and alleviating compassion fatigue through self-care: an educational workshop for nurses. J Holist Nurs. 2018;36(4):304–17.

40. Alexander GK, Rollins K, Walker D, Wong L, Pennings J. Yoga for self-care and burnout prevention among nurses. Workplace Health Saf. 2015;63(10):462–70.

41. Ali G, Snowden M. SOPHIE (self-exploration through ontological, phenomenological, humanistic, ideological and existential expressions): a mentoring framework. In: Snowden M, Halsall J, editors. Mentorship, leadership, and research. International perspectives on social policy, administration, and practice. Cham: Springer; 2019.

42. Bakker A, Sanz-Vergel A. Weekly work engagement and flourishing: the role of hindrance and challenge job demands. J Vocat Behav. 2013;83(3):397–409. https://doi.org/10.1016/j.jvb.2013.06.008.

43. Bamonti PM, Keelan CM, Larson N, Mentrikoski JM, Randall CL, Sly SK, McNeil DW, et al. Promoting ethical behavior by cultivating a culture of self-care during graduate training: a call to action. Training Educ Profession Psychol. 2014;8(4):253.

44. Bartram T, et al. Do perceived high performance work systems influence the relationship between emotional labour, burnout and intention to leave? A study of Australian nurses. J Adv Nurs. 2012;68(7):1567–78.

45. Barss K. T.R.U.S.T.: an affirming model for inclusive spiritual care. J Holist Nurs. 2012;30(1):24–34.

46. Beaumont E, Durkin M, Hollins Martin C, Carson J. Measuring relationships between self-compassion, compassion fatigue, burnout and well-being in student counsellors and student cognitive behavioural psychotherapists: a quantitative survey. Couns Psychother Res. 2018;16(1):15–23. https://doi.org/10.1002/capr.12054.

47. Björkström ME, Athlin EE, Johansson IS. Nurses' development of professional self—from being a nursing student in a baccalaureate programme to an experienced nurse. J Clin Nurs. 2008;1710:1380–139.

48. Bloom. YSHP. 2018. https://yourspiritualhealth.org/.

49. Bostwick A, Kerry A, Mills K. Clinical pocket reference: fundamental care: a person centred approach. 2015. www.clinicalpocketreference.com.

50. Brown B. The gifts of imperfection. Minnesota: Hazelden; 2010.

51. Brown S, Whichello R, Price S. The impact of resiliency on nurse burnout: an integrative literature review. Medsurg Nurs. 2018;27(6):349–78.

52. Funk L, Peters S, Roger K. Caring about dying persons and their families: interpretation, practice and emotional labour. Health Social Care Commun. 2017;26(4):519–26. https://doi.org/10.1111/hsc.12559.

53. Gentry E. Fighting compassion fatigue and burnout by building emotional resilience. J Oncol Navigat Survivor. 2018;9(12):532–5.

54. Goleman D. Emotional intelligence: why it can matter more than IQ. New York: Bantam Books; 1995.

55. Griffiths J, Speed S, Horne M, Keeley P. A caring professional attitude': what service users and carers seek in graduate nurses and the challenge for educators. Nurse Educ Today. 2012;32(2012):121–7. https://doi.org/10.1016/j.nedt.2011.06.005.

56. Heffernan M. Wilful blindness. New York: Simon and Schuster; 2011.

57. Henson J. When compassion is lost. Medsurg Nurs. 2017;26:139–42.

58. Hofmeyer A, Toffoli L, Vernon R, Taylor R, Klopper HC, Coetzee SK, Fontaine D. Teaching compassionate care to nursing students in a digital learning and teaching environment. Collegian. 2018;25(3):307–12.

59. Hunsaker S, Chen H, Maughan D, Heaston S. Factors that influence the development of compassion fatigue. J Nurs Scholarsh. 2014;47(2):186–94. https://doi.org/10.1111/jnu.12122.

60. Jenkins R. Social identity. London: Routledge; 2008.

61. Johnson M, Cowin LS. Professional identity and nursing: contemporary theoretical developments and future research challenges. Int Nurs Rev. 2012;59(4):562–9.

62. Kravits K, McAllister-Black R, Grant M, Kirk C. Self-care strategies for nurses: a psychoeducational intervention for stress reduction and the prevention of burnout. Appl Nurs Res. 2010;23(3):130–8.

63. McCabe R, Nowak M, Mullen S. Nursing careers: what motivated nurses to choose their profession? Aust Bull Labour. 2005;31(4):321–49.

64. McCance T, Slater P, McCormack B. Using the caring dimensions inventory as an indicator. J Clin Nurs. 2009;18:409–17. https://doi.org/10.1111/j.1365-2702.2008.02466.x.

65. McCormack B, McCance T. Person-centred practice in nursing and health care theory and practice. 2nd ed. Hoboken, NJ: Wiley; 2017.

66. McMahon R. Therapeutic nursing—theory, issues and practice. In: Pearson A, editor. Nursing as therapy. Cheltenham: Stanley Thornes; 1998.

67. McSherry W, Jamieson S. An online survey of nurses' perceptions of spirituality and spiritual care. J Clin Nurs. 2011;20:1757–67. https://doi.org/10.1111/j.1365-2702.2010.03547.x.

68. Mayo Clinic. 2018. https://www.mayoclinic.org/healthy-lifestyle/stress-management/in-depth/exercise-and-stress/art-20044469.

69. Mills J, Wand T, Fraser JA. Examining self-care, self-compassion and compassion for others: a cross-sectional survey of palliative care nurses and doctors. Int J Palliat Nurs. 2018;24(1):4–11.

70. Muetzel P. Therapeutic nursing, in primary nursing: nursing in the Burford and Oxford nursing development units. Beckenham: Croom Helm; 1988.

71. Pollard J. Authenticity and inauthenticity. In: van Deurzen E, Arnold Baker C, editors. Existential perspectives on human issues—a handbook for therapeutic practice. New York: Palgrave; 2005.

72. Rolheiser R. The restless heart: finding our spiritual home in times of loneliness. New York: Double Day; 2004.

73. Routson J. Emotional intelligence: an essential skill for nurses. 2010. https://www.healthecar-
eers.com/article/career/emotional-intelligence-an-essential-skill-for-nurses.

74. Rushton C, Batcheller J, Schroeder K, Donohue P. Burnout and resilience among nurses practicing in high-intensity settings. Am J Crit Care. 2015;24(5):412–20. https://doi.org/10.4037/
ajcc20155291.

75. Schaubroeck J, Jones JR. Antecedents of emotional labour dimensions and moderators of their
effects on physical symptoms. J Organ Behav. 2000;21:163–83.

76. Sergeant J, Laws-Chapman C. Creating a positive workplace culture. Nurs Manage.
2012;18:14–9.

77. Sheppard K. Compassion fatigue: are you at risk? Am Nurse Today. 2016;11:53–5. https://
www.americannursetoday.com. Accessed December 2019.

78. Schmid P. Authenticity: the person as his or her own author. Dialogical and ethical perspectives on therapy as an encounter relationship and beyond. In: Wyatt G, editor. Congruence.
Ross-on-Wye: Llongarron; 2001. p. 201–16.

79. Smith-Trudeau P. Moving from compassion fatigue to self-compassion. Vermont Nurse
Connect. 2019;22(3):1–3.

80. Snowden A, Telfer IJ, Kelly EK, Bunniss S, Mowat H. 'I was able to talk about what was on my
mind'. The operationalisation of person centred care. Scot J Healthc Chaplain. 2013;16:14–24.

81. Snowden A, Gibbon A, Grant R. What is the impact of chaplaincy in primary care? The GP perspective. Health Social Care Chaplain. 2018;6(2):200–14. https://doi.org/10.1558/hscc.34709.

82. Snowden A, Telfer I. The Scottish PROM. In: Kelly E, Swinton J, editors. Chaplaincy and the
soul of health and social care: fostering spiritual wellbeing in emerging paradigms of care.
London: Jessica Kingsley; 2020. p. 67–89.

83. Stamm BH. The concise ProQOL manual. 2nd ed. Pocatello, ID: ProQOL.org; 2012.

84. Stress Research Institute. Stress Research Institute. 2010. http://www.stressforskning.su.se/
pub/jsp/polopoly.jsp?d=4746. 3 Socialstyrelsen.

85. Wadhill-Goad S. Stress, fatigue and burnout in nursing. J Radiol Nurs. 2013;38:44–6. https://
doi.org/10.1016/j.jradnu.2018.10.

Suggested Reading

Brown B. Daring greatly: how the courage to be vulnerable transforms the way we live, love, parent, and lead. New York: Gotham Books; 2012.

Gawande A. Being mortal: medicine and what matters in the end. New York: Metropolitan Books,
Henry Holt; 2014.

Hayes SC, Strosahl KD, Wilson KG. Acceptance and commitment therapy: the process and practice of mindful change. 2nd ed. New York: The Guilford Press; 2012.

Rogers CR. On becoming a person: a therapist's view of psychotherapy. Boston: Houghton
Mifflin; 1995.

Chapter 5
Competence 1: Intrapersonal Spirituality and Its Impact on Person-Centred Spiritual Care

René van Leeuwen, Gørill Haugan, Melanie Rogers, Åsa Roxberg, Joanna Zolnierz, and Anto Čartolovni

---

Learning Objectives

This chapter will enable you:

1. To understand the impact of intrapersonal spirituality on a person's health and well-being across the lifespan and how this impacts the provision of person- centred care (knowledge).

R. van Leeuwen (✉)
Viaa Christian University of Applied Sciences, Zwolle, The Netherlands
e-mail: r.vanleeuwen@viaa.nl

G. Haugan
Norwegian University of Science and Technology, Trondheim, Norway

Faculty of Nursing and Health Science, Nord University, Bodø, Norway
e-mail: gorill.haugan@ntnu.no

M. Rogers
University of Huddersfield, Huddersfield, UK
e-mail: M.Rogers@hud.ac.uk

Å. Roxberg
Caring Sciences, University West, Trollhättan, Sweden

VID University, Stavanger, Norway
e-mail: asa.roxberg@hv.se

J. Zolnierz
Interfaculty Centre for Didactics, Medical University of Lublin, Lublin, Poland

A. Čartolovni
Digital Healthcare Ethics Laboratory (Digit-HeaL), Catholic University of Croatia, Zagreb, Croatia

Faculty of Health Sciences, University of Hull, Hull, UK
e-mail: anto.cartolovni@unicath.hr

© Springer Nature Switzerland AG 2021
W. McSherry et al. (eds.), *Enhancing Nurses' and Midwives' Competence in Providing Spiritual Care*, https://doi.org/10.1007/978-3-030-65888-5_5

2. To reflect meaningfully upon your own values and beliefs and how they may differ from others.
3. To learn how to take care of oneself whilst providing spiritual care (skills).
4. To be open and respectful to individuals' diverse expressions of spirituality (attitude).

5.1   Introduction

This chapter has paid attention to the competence of intrapersonal spirituality. From a patients' perspective, intrapersonal spirituality relates to the impact of an individuals' spirituality on his or her health and well-being. From the perspective of nurses and midwives, intrapersonal spirituality relates to the impact of one's own values and beliefs in providing spiritual care. Nurses and midwives should show willingness to explore one's own and their patients/clients' personal, religious and spiritual beliefs. The EPICC spiritual care competences are clear about that. It is important whilst doing this to be open and respectful to others' diverse expressions of spirituality. The intrapersonal competence asks for meaningful reflection upon one's own values and beliefs and the recognition that can differ from other people. In this chapter, different elements of the intrapersonal competence will be discussed. Firstly, the context of intrapersonal spirituality will be explored by emphasising the holistic approach in health care, its position within the nurse/midwife–patient relationship and the importance of the consciousness of one's own values and beliefs. How intrapersonal spirituality is operationalised in nursing and midwifery practice, based on the concepts of attention, presence, availability and vulnerability will be discussed. Through a combination of practice-based scenarios and reflective exercises, the reader will cover the key elements outlined in Competence 2 (Box 5.1) within the EPICC Spiritual Care Education Standard [1]. The chapter ends with a practical guideline for the exploration of one's own spirituality by use of the FICA model [2].

Box 5.1: Intrapersonal Spirituality

Is aware of the importance of spirituality on health and well-being		
Knowledge (cognitive)	Skills (functional)	Attitudes (behavioural)
– Understands the concept of spirituality – Can explain the impact of spirituality on a person's health and well-being across the lifespan for oneself and others. – Understands the impact of one's own values and beliefs in providing spiritual care	– Reflects meaningfully upon one's own values and beliefs and recognises that these may be different from other persons' – Takes care of oneself	– Willing to explore one's own and individuals' personal, religious and spiritual beliefs – Is open and respectful to persons' diverse expressions of spirituality

This chapter starts with some brief images from healthcare practice that relate to the intrapersonal aspects of spirituality and can impact our thoughts and feelings. Questions like these: 'What does a patient still live for?' 'How can someone even live in this situation?' or 'How do these situations affect my own personal thoughts and emotions?' are all important questions to reflect upon.

'Angela is 19 years old and about to deliver her first baby in 6 weeks' time. The baby was not planned, and her pregnancy physiologically has not been easy. There haven't been any major complications, the baby seems healthy, but it is an anxious time for her. She asks herself a lot of questions about motherhood and raising a child: 'Will I be a good mother, what does it ask from me? The relationship with her boyfriend is problematic. He has told her that he is not ready to become a father'.

'A terminal patient has three children, aged six, four and two. She knows she will be leaving them behind, and this is painful and difficult for her. It has broken her emotionally. As a nurse I found this very difficult, because she would not let any of the staff in to support her with her thoughts and feelings. I found this very difficult. I feel helpless. I can see her struggling with fundamental questions of life, but what can I do? I want to help her!'

'I am not religious and because of that I sometimes feel some resistance within myself when I care for someone with a religious faith. For example, I met with a young 29 years old cancer patient. She was a strong Christian. She talked about it often and told me that she is praying a lot. She told me that prayer gives her a lot of support. I found this very difficult to understand and this in turn makes it difficult for me to relate to her'. How should I manage this situation?'

'Sometimes it is too much for me. I see patients suffer and I want to cry. Sometimes when I reflect with colleagues on certain situations, I do cry. Is this ok or do I have to handle my emotions in a different way? It isn't easy not to show emotions. Is it alright to share and show my own feelings to the patient?'

'At the moment my own life is not so easy to live. I experience a lot of stress in my work and in my private life. There is a lot at stake. My first experience in clinical practice as a student nurse was very challenging. I nursed lots of older patients who appeared to have nothing left to live for, I couldn't change my perspective on this. I asked myself: "What do they live for?" Is this my future as a nurse? How can I give my patients more meaning and purpose when they are coming to the end of their lives? How can I change my perspective?'

Before continuing studying this chapter, reflect on the above vignettes by considering the following questions:

- Do you recognise one or more of these situations from your own practice/experience?
- What questions and emotions arose within you?
- How did you handle that situation?
- What are in your opinion important aspects of intrapersonal spirituality in healthcare?

5.2 The Context of Intrapersonal Spirituality

Paying attention to one's own spirituality by relying on the holistic view of a human being is fundamental to good practice and has significant benefits for the nurse/midwife–patient relationship. It enables nurses and midwives to view their patient or client as a person with a unique life story and unique views of his or her life. That persons' intrapersonal spirituality impacts also the nurses' and midwife's own values and beliefs and his or her relationship with the patient. It necessitates a person-centred relationship which will be discussed later in the chapter. Working in this way the nurses' and midwifes' consciousness of his or her own values and beliefs will be emphasised.

5.2.1 Spirituality and Spiritual Care Within the Holistic Understanding of Healthcare

Nursing and midwifery are grounded in the holistic understanding of health [3], which considers spirituality to be a vital aspect of people's health and well-being [4, 5]. Individuals are seen as a whole with a physical, mental, social and spiritual/existential dimension. Nursing and midwifery students are presented to this holistic understanding of health consisting of the four above-mentioned dimensions. However, in this way, we theoretically split humans into four, which is contradictory. This picture of a human being divided into four parts, dimensions, is only theoretical. Figure 5.1 illustrates that human beings comprise these four dimensions but does also include a circulating red dotted line. Even though we theoretically claim that there are different dimensions, individuals are still a unit of integrated dimensions, physical, mental, social and spiritual/existential, which are interrelated and influence each other. An interaction between the parts or levels in the whole are steadily going on, controlled via the brain [6].

Hence, patients and clients are unique and indivisible physical-psycho-social-spiritual entities where body, soul and spirit are integrated and constantly interact

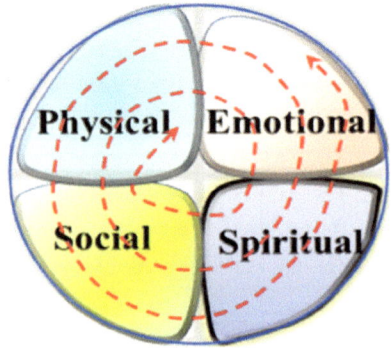

Fig. 5.1 The wholeness of man involving a physical, psychological, social and spiritual dimension, inter-related by means of a steadily interaction between the levels/dimensions. © Haugan [8]

with each other. That is, the human experiences, expectations, thoughts and feelings 99
are spiritual, emotional and physiological states or biochemical conditions in the 100
body, with subsequent bodily consequences, thereby impacting the rest of the per- 101
son [3]. Research has shown and shows ever more clearly that there are connections 102
(interaction) between the spirit, soul (the mind, our thoughts, feelings and experi- 103
ences) and the body in the development of most diseases, ailments and suffering. 104
Patients' and clients' emotions are biochemical realities in their bodies; the emo- 105
tions have no other place to be. Candace Pert [6], an internationally recognised 106
stress researcher, has shown that the brain 'talks' to the immune cell system using 107
'messenger cells' called neuropeptides or transmitters. When the brain interprets 108
emotions such as fear, anger or sadness, all the immune cells are told about this 109
interpretation. Pert ([6], p. 27–32) describes this process as 'bits of the brain floating 110
around the body'. Simply put, we can say that our spirit, the emotions and thoughts 111
'float around the body', materialised as peptides (protein molecules) and a myriad 112
of complex chemical and physiological processes. In this light, the importance of 113
spirituality within the healthcare contexts is evident and well defined [7]. Spiritual 114
care is about supporting patients' and clients' search and expression of what gives 115
their life meaning, purpose as well as facilitating their connectedness to self, others, 116
nature and for some people a transcendent being, such as God. 117

Recent studies have shown by using structural equation modelling (SEM analy- 118
sis) that how nursing home patients perceive the interaction with their nurses, sig- 119
nificantly impacts on their perceived joy-of-life [9], meaning-in-life, sense of 120
coherence, hope, self-transcendence, anxiety and depression [8]. 121

5.2.2   *Intrapersonal Spirituality Embedded Within the Nurse/* 122
Midwife–Patient Relationship 123

By listening to patients'/clients' feelings, taking them seriously as well as 124
respecting and affirming the person for who they are often mediates the interac- 125
tion/experience of meaningful contact, self-transcendence and meaning-in-life 126
[8, 10]. Both meaning and self-transcendence have shown a significant impact 127
on anxiety and depression, as well as on physical, emotional, social, functional 128
and spiritual well-being [8]. Spiritual care is embedded in the nurse/midwife– 129
patient interaction, by relational qualities that support and facilitate the human 130
spirit. The experience of trust, respect, being understood, listened to and taken 131
seriously, being seen and recognised as the person you are, nurtures patient's 132
and clients spirit and thereby their body, enhancing their recovery and health. 133
Nurses and midwives represent an important resource of human contact. In the 134
face of serious illness, trauma, losses, death, life-changing events and transi- 135
tions in life, such as pregnancy/delivery or retirement, individuals' vulnerability 136
increases [11]. This is especially true in relationship with those in power, such 137
as nurses, midwives and other healthcare professionals, who have power for 138
both good and bad. 139

5.2.3   The Importance of Consciousness and Impact of One's Own Spirituality

The nurse/midwife–patient interaction is a twofold process where not only patient/ clients receive and nurses/midwives give, but nurses/midwives also receive by becoming aware of the importance of their own spirituality (intrapersonal) and connectedness and value to others. This awareness further manifests in the form of the existential inquiry about getting to know yourself. The interest in human reality started in the antiquity period by wondering about what kind of being is a human and does it differentiate from other living and non-living beings. In ancient Greece, one of the famous expressions was 'know thyself', which was ascribed at the doorway of the Apollo's temple in Delphi. Although it was a commonly used phrase in Ancient Greece, often its authorship is mistakenly ascribed to Socrates as one of the greatest thinkers at that time. Getting to know yourself summarises the synergy between thinking (epistemology) and being (ontology), referring for most of the thinkers at that time the relationship between the finite and infinity, or transcendence and immanence. For Greek philosophers, the human body is a starting point in inquiry about themselves, as they perceived human beings to be not only biological matter but also spiritual having a soul defined and differentiated humans from other living creatures. For Socrates, getting to know yourself was only possible through his maieutic (midwifery) method, which consisted in establishing a dialogue between himself (who asks the question) and the soul (who answers). The dialogue between himself as something finite and immanent and the soul as something infinite and transcendent represents for Socrates a true nature of human existence. This dialogue served for Socrates as not only for finding the right answers to the burning questions but also the existential worth in it by stating 'an unexamined life is not worth living' ([12], p. 128). Therefore, if we want to recognise and respond to the spiritual needs of others actively, we need to be familiar with our own spiritual life by examining and familiarising with it.

The pursuit for the existential meaning steers each individual to find a meaning in their life by verging towards their inner self and asking questions about themselves, their existence, their finitude and whether anything does or does not exist external to them. Some people find their answers to part of the questions within themselves in their awareness of being-in-the-world, whilst others seek answers beyond their awareness of being-in-the-world in the infinite i.e. in transcendence. This desire to acquire the knowledge about ourselves is a special kind of drive for one of the famous continental philosophers Emanuel Lévinas, an essential characteristic of human beings who are always turned towards otherness [13]. The attitudes of seeking, desiring and questioning represents the best environment for the revelation of the otherness, and the otherness represents a form of face-to-face relationship where every face we encounter is a face of the other. As for the philosophers, in the antiquity period, including Lévinas, the human body is essential in this self-knowing approach, because the body is not only a 'chunk of matter', nor it is an expression of the soul, but it represents an event of the infinite, demanding a responsibility towards other [14]. Lévinas and Cohen [15] also suggested that in a face-to-face encounter, the other i.e. our neighbour, by revealing itself as being different, vulnerable and exposed shifts this encounter from our own existential confirmation into ethical call. The face-to-face encounter of the patients does not only mean the affirmation of the professional role that healthcare personnel has, but the affirmation of the needs that the patient/client (other) posses. This represents a starting point of our awareness about responsibility towards other (our neighbour, patient/client) through which we do not only recognise their existence but we also give some kind of appreciation of the presence of the infinite in them, and through this appreciation, we reassure our existence of being human as spiritual beings. This awareness of the responsibility of the other and recognition the infinite in our patients/clients emerge every time when we approach them with the dignified care. Therefore, this openness represents a relational aspect of a human in its ability to be faced by the other human being and by the infinite, as something residing outside of our own being. Furthermore, this openness towards the infinite as inherently dwelled in human nature represents a space for revelation, transcendence on which many religions rely. Therefore, this openness towards something and the ability to relate to it, even going beyond our human reason and capability to understand in reality represents who we are. Human spiritual beings who always stand in relation with other human beings, and from this relational responsibility towards other we gain our self-awareness and knowledge about the relation with the other (the infinite). This relational aspect of spirituality represents an inter-relational aspect that especially comes forth in nursing and midwifery, where encountering patients/clients with their different life situations/states awakens interest among nurses/midwives to consider more about meaning of their own life/existence and spirituality in order better to understand and answer to the patient's/client's spiritual needs. This relational aspect reaffirms the fact that spirituality in nursing/midwifery dwells from the practice and is deeply endowed in the practice shaping it in the form of a more person-centred care.

Intrapersonal spirituality also refers to intrapersonal values, like what is most important for each person, such as relations to oneself, family, friends, work, things nature, art and culture, ethics and morals, and life itself [7]. These values embrace spirituality as the very core enabling the provision of genuine spiritual care. The definition of spirituality that was introduced in the introduction of this book, includes some important concepts that may provide guidance as to what the intrapersonal values are and mean. It says that spirituality is dynamic, which means that the intrapersonal values of spiritual care are a force, not ascertain once and for all. It changes according to the other person in the care moment and adheres to the person cared for express and/or seek meaning, purpose and transcendence. Personal values can be recognised and understood by nurses and midwives when they have an understanding of spirituality. It is important to recognise that this differs from religion or cultural belief, and it is not necessary for the nurse/midwife to share their patients'/clients' beliefs in order to integrate interpersonal values into the care offered. With that intrapersonal competence follows an understanding of what it means to seek meaning, purpose and transcendence. The way to connect to the

228 moment to self, to others, to nature, to the significant and/or the sacred, as men-
229 tioned in the definition of spirituality, is a matter of being competent to understand
230 the other in a trying life situation and what it means to be human [7]. Referring to
231 Anne Bogart, an American film director who maintained that 'to truly be a bearer of
232 an ethos is to be completely open for the unknown, the unpredictable, and that
233 which no one can control, allowing one to meet reality as it actually is' [16]. For the
234 nurses and midwifes to have this openness means to be aware of the own vulnerabil-
235 ity in order to be able to sense the vulnerability of the other [17]. To be open to one
236 another is a way of mediating humanity since both the patient and the caregiver are
237 part of what it means to be human [18]. To dare to explore ones' own vulnerability
238 is therefore an essential part of developing excellent nursing care. It does not mean
239 to expose yourself fully but to be able to develop a true two-way communication
240 based on openness for the uniqueness of oneself and the uniqueness of the other. It
241 is also the path to a true presence, which is the essence of a caring consolation [19].

> **Reflection**
> This paragraph explores the context of intrapersonal spirituality within nurs-
> ing and midwifery.
>   You can reflect on this by answering and discussing the following questions:
>   – How do you integrate the holistic perspective in your nursing/midwifery
> care and ensure that your patient/client is recognised as a unique person.
>   – You are entering a hospital room with a patient who is turning his back
> against you. The patient has been admitted the day before and it is your first
> meeting with him. The sense mediated from this response is emptiness and
> loneliness. Reflect on how you best approach this patient to alleviate his
> suffering.
>   – What do you think is meant by the relational aspect of spiritual care? Do
> you recognise the face-to-face encounter as awakening of the responsibility
> for caring for the patient/client? How can you recognise that in your own
> care giving?

242 ## 5.3   The Essence of Intrapersonal Spirituality in Nursing
243 ##   and Midwifery Practice

244 This section discusses how intrapersonal spirituality impacts the nurse/midwife–
245 patient relationship through being present (prescencing), attentive, available and
246 vulnerable. It shows that the nurse and midwife cannot overlook themselves but put
247 himself or herself in the 'relational spotlight' in order to provide spiritual care.

5.3.1 Presence and Attention   248

Nurses' and midwives' spiritual competence involves attentional and influencing   249
skills [20]. Nurses' attention and presence are the leading 'tools'. Good nurse/mid-   250
wife–patient interaction is based on attention-related skills. Nurses and midwives   251
consciously use and regulate their attention; that is, what one sees, hears, feels,   252
smells, senses and thinks during the interaction with the patient/client. Consideration 253
of what are you paying attention to or where do you direct your attention can   254
improve the interaction.   255

During spiritual care, the nurse/midwife–patient/client interaction requires   256
awareness skills that are based on an active and open reception presence. Identified   257
that a sensory presence during which you look to see and listen to hear in order to   258
welcome and attend to what you see and hear is a way to improve the interaction of   259
those being cared for. Utilising sensory presence in this way enables the patient's   260
inner world, representing who he/she is right now, to be welcomed and accepted;   261
that is his/her experiences, emotions and thoughts are accepted as they are. Working   262
in this way leads to trust being established because the patient/client will experience 263
being taken seriously, being seen and heard. This experience promotes well-being   264
and health among those being cared for. This way of working also creates a com-   265
mon understanding of what is at stake right now for the patient/client; what do they   266
think, feel and experience? These emotions and experiences should be given atten-   267
tion and understood by the nurse of midwife in order for the patient/client to become 268
a fully recognised person who is viewed as whole and integrated being, a spiritual   269
being [8].   270

Attention skills include the nurse/midwife noting the patient/client's choice of   271
words, the volume, tone and power of the voice, as well as rhythm of expression,   272
tempo (fast, slow, pauses), non-verbal expressions such as a sigh, breath, gaze,   273
facial expression, skin colour, posture, congruence and authenticity. These cues pro- 274
vide a wealth of information about the patients/clients' well-being for those who are   275
aware [8]. These cues are crucial in spiritual care which is more about experience   276
and feeling than thinking. The instrument of your attention is yourself and what you   277
see, hear, feel and sense. These skills need the nurse/midwife to be in contact with   278
one's inner self with a focus of attention fully on the patient/client. Therefore, it is 279
important to notice whether undue attention is paid to something else or if there is   280
any lack of attention to something that should be given your attention.   281

A patient who dares to share with you about her feeling of loneliness represents   282
an example illustrating this point. She is crying; what are you paying attention to?   283
The factual content about her loneliness? Or the emotional expression of crying?   284
What are you doing? Are you listening? Do you explore what this is about? Or do   285
you start to comfort? There is no one facet. However, taking time to listen and   286
explore, allowing the patient room and space to become clear to themselves will facili- 287
tate spiritual well-being and health, and will be more soothing than well-intentioned 288

289 comfort. Often, nurses and midwives' attempts to comfort become more of a strat-
290 egy that maintains the suffering, rather than helping to relieve it. For example,
291 focusing on what this woman is saying about being lonely instead of focusing on
292 her crying can, paradoxically, cause this lady to feel overlooked, rejected and thus
293 feel even more lonely. Attention to the matter and a cognitive understanding of its
294 content is usually not enough. Attention to emotional expressions is very important
295 in ensuring the true meaning of what the patient/client in your care is under-
296 stood fully.
297   Spiritual care rests on nurse and midwives' listening abilities and their capability
298 to create rapport; i.e. identifying and caring about the 'what is' in the experience of
299 the patient. In every patient interaction relationship, nurses and midwives are depen-
300 dent on their attention skills which is key to making clear what is at stake in the
301 patient's life just now. Being aware of cues and hints that give useful information is
302 an important aspect of spiritual care. Moreover, nurse/midwife–patient interactions,
303 and thus spiritual care, are about sustaining professional boundaries between nurse/
304 midwife and patient/client so that respect and dignity are maintained. Empathic
305 listening providing unconditional acceptance, tenderness, recognition and empathy
306 creates experiences of acceptance and respect and can lead to changes—perhaps
307 especially in relation to self and inner processes. Nursing literature also acknowl-
308 edges skills such as interpretation, confrontation, giving advice, recommendation or
309 instruction which represent even more direct impact when providing spiritual care.
310 Both influencing and attentional skills signify the use of power and impact, which
311 are part of all relationships between nurses/midwives and their patients/clients.
312 Openly or hidden, power, influence and authority are always there. Thus, patient/
313 client interactions require that healthcare professionals are perceptive of one's
314 power and how to use it for positive impacts. The attention is not about if or whether
315 power is being used, but how it is used. Wanting the other well, unconditional
316 acceptance, authenticity and warmth are always the foundation on which health-
317 promoting interaction must be based. Nurses and midwives are present whilst per-
318 forming the various tasks in collaboration with the patient/client which determines
319 the experienced care quality and is fundamental to patient's well-being. Nursing
320 studies have displayed that the nurse–patient interaction significantly influences
321 older adults' anxiety, depression, hope, meaning and self-transcendence, as well as
322 joy-of-life and the experience of belonging and connectedness [8, 9]. This means
323 that by means of awareness, tenderness, empathic listening and influencing skills,
324 the nurse–patient interaction can be used to competently influence vulnerable indi-
325 vidual's well-being and health, spiritually/existentially, physically, psychologically,
326 and socially. Nurses and midwives '*being in the doing*' can influence patients' mul-
327 tidimensional well-being.
328   For nurses and midwives to be able to connect fully with those in their care,
329 intrapersonal spirituality is fundamental. Yet, intrapersonal spirituality may feel like
330 a philosophical concept that cannot be easily understood or expressed through one's
331 work. A framework to develop and sustain intrapersonal spirituality and support

nurses to provide spiritual care is presented here as a tangible way to integrate spiri-   332
tuality into clinical practice [21, 22]. The framework is based upon the concepts of   333
availability and vulnerability, adapted and validated for nursing and applicable also   334
to midwifery. The origins of the concepts derive from the Northumbria Community,   335
a Celtic monastic community [23]. It is a privilege and honour as nurses and mid-   336
wives to be able to connect and walk alongside those in our care in the midst of   337
stress, illness and distress. It is during these times that patients/clients often express   338
their fears, anxieties and struggles to us. We have the ability and choice at these   339
times to connect deeply and provide support and comfort (intrapersonal spirituality/   340
person-centred care) or to carry out our work in a more mechanistic task-   341
oriented way.   342

In relationship to intrapersonal spirituality, availability and vulnerability can be   343
integrated and practiced by nurses and midwives to build the own understanding of   344
their personal spirituality and the spiritual needs of those in their care. It enables   345
nurses and midwives to be fully present and provide holistic care in an authentic   346
person-centred way. By living and working in a way which embraces availability   347
and vulnerability nurses and midwives can develop meaningful relationships recog-   348
nising the importance of maintaining a nurse–patient relationship based on trust,   349
honesty and acceptance. Thorup et al. [24] and [25] all have explored aspects of   350
availability and vulnerability in their work, suggesting that nurses' ability to care for   351
others necessitates a depth of love and connection which derives from an under-   352
standing of their vocation, their own personal values and attributes. Availability and   353
vulnerability involve connecting with others as fellow human beings through an   354
authentic reflective and an altruistic approach to nursing and midwifery.   355

Reflection
Think about a situation when you felt really present with one of your patients/
clients. Answer the following questions:
   – How did you experience the contact with the patient/client as a
unique human being?
   – What were your emotions in this situation?
   – Can you think about a situation where your sensory presence was
your main tool?
   Do you recognise a situation that a patient dares to share with you their
feelings of loneliness, about not or barely being connected to anyone or any
what? If so, answer the following questions:
   – What do you want to pay attention to? The factual content about her
loneliness? Or the emotional expression of crying?
   – What are your thoughts and what do you feel?
   – How do you use your attention skills?

5.4 Availability

Availability is a concept that will be familiar to nurses and midwives, especially physical availability where day-to-day care is provided. This in itself can be practiced in several ways. Nurses and midwives can provide care as a task with little interaction and connection with their patients/clients, or they can provide the care holistically in a way that respects and values spirituality. For example, maintaining dignity whilst carrying out aspect of care which could leave a patient/client feeling uncomfortable or embarrassed. There are two other important aspects of availability that nurses and midwives have a choice whether to integrate into their care, emotional and vocational availability, these are integral to intrapersonal spirituality as they necessitate connection with our patients/clients as fellow human beings. Availability in all these ways is illustrated as principles of availability to self, to others and to the community.

Availability to self enables the nurse/midwife to understand and reflect on their own attitudes, values and beliefs. The key to this principle is self-acceptance and a willingness to embrace one's own spirituality. Reflection on personal spirituality involves consideration of what gives hope, meaning, purpose and direction in life. For many nurses and midwives, this involves the vocational element of their work. Availability to others is a choice that involves more than just nursing tasks. It involves welcoming people into your care by offering your time, acceptance and understanding. It necessitates fully present and listening attentively to the needs verbally and non-verbally of those in our care. Understanding the patients/clients' personal, religion and spiritual needs and integrating these into the care provided is fundamental to care and recovery. Availability to community is the choice to adapt and develop your clinical practice in response to the needs of those in your 'community'. This is related to the individual needs of the clinical area for example the needs of the elderly, patients undergoing surgery, etc.

Availability stems from the acceptance and understanding of ourselves in addition to the commitment to nursing as a vocation. Developing relationships with ourselves, others and the community around us based upon authenticity and compassion enables the nurse/midwife to be fully present. It is recognised that working in this way develops trust and assists healing and recovery [26].

5.5 Vulnerability

Embracing vulnerability in a clinical setting may appear more contentious as it may be perceived by some as a weakness or leading to the possibility of being hurt [17]. However, being vulnerable personally and with others leads to more open, honest and authentic relationships [27]. The principles of vulnerability include vulnerability to self, to others and the community.

Vulnerability to self includes the acknowledgement of the vulnerability of nurs- 394
ing/midwifery and the reality that you can never 'know it all'. As we begin to rec- 395
ognise that our patients/clients do not expect us to know everything and desire a 396
relationship based on honesty and respect we can enter into relationships based 397
upon a willingness to be with others as a fellow human being with a recognition that 398
we are all fallible. Working in this way includes an element of risk of being misun- 399
derstood or too open with our patients/clients. However, research identified that 400
demonstrating vulnerability has significant positive effect on relationships and trust 401
[24, 27]. 402

Vulnerability with others enables clinical practice to be more authentic. It 403
includes being fully present and being able to acknowledge our own mistakes and 404
limitations. It involves accepting that we do not know it all or have all the answers 405
and being able to share our uncertainty with patients revealing our openness, hon- 406
esty and transparency and willingness to be human. 407

Vulnerability to the community includes the willingness to advocate for those in 408
your care questioning authority where necessary, keeping with the interests of your 409
patients/clients at the centre of care. 410

Vulnerability impacts our ability to connect with others authentically. Many 411
nurses/midwives may have been taught the importance of emotional distance from 412
their patients/clients. However, working in this way negates human connection. 413
Being vulnerable is about authentic relationships within the professional and ethical 414
boundaries of our profession. It is about being human in how we connect and inter- 415
act and is as Brown [27] states a risk we have to take if we want to experience 416
connection. 417

> **Reflection**
> – Think about a time when you have been away of integrating availability
> into your own practice. Reflect on how this occurred and how it affected your
> connection to the patient/client?
> – Reflect on the following statement: *'Being vulnerable in your work
> as a nurse/midwife may never be perceived as weakness, but always as being
> authentic in relationship to the patient/client'*.
> – Describe a spiritual care situation from your clinical practice where
> you showed your vulnerability. What happened and how did it work out?

5.6 Discover Your Personal Intrapersonal Spirituality   418

An extremely important task facing a professionally prepared nurse and midwife is 419
caring for one's own spiritual dimension. The attitude of caring for your own spiri- 420
tuality and religiosity should be shaped especially at the stage of professional prepa- 421
ration for nursing and midwifery. The teaching strategies and tools developed and 422
described by the participants of the EPICC Project, collected in the EPICC Toolbox, 423

424 are great knowledge compendium. On the official website of the project, dedicated
425 to the issues of Intrapersonal spirituality, you can find a detailed description of up to
426 17 educational strategies. Practical exercises encouraging nursing and midwifery
427 students to self-reflection, finding sources of their beliefs and define their value
428 system, are to realise that the spirituality of the nurse/midwife is an integral part of
429 her/his professional work. The 'availability and vulnerability' model described by
430 Rogers in this chapter is an example for that.
431   Just as their own system of values and beliefs are an important source of spiritual
432 strength and affect motivation to work, so spiritual distress can destabilise the func-
433 tioning of a person in all areas of their life, including the field of professional work.
434 Effective spiritual care and self-awareness are therefore essential skills for a nurse
435 and midwife. Understanding the role of proper care for one's own spirituality initi-
436 ated the process of change in curricula, but also led to the development of many
437 tools to facilitate taking care of one's own spirituality by already practicing nurses
438 and midwives. It is worth emphasising that in addition to support groups, fully pro-
439 fessional pastoral care programs, a wide range of training and lectures as well as
440 courses for nurses and midwives, many tools have also been created to facilitate
441 quick self-diagnosis and analysis of one's spiritual history. Tools from The Spiritual
442 History Tool group, whose names are usually an acronym, are very effective, because
443 with a few questions they help assess your own spirituality, and their use does not
444 require specialised knowledge or special instrumentation [28]. Often used tool in
445 this group is 'FICA for Self-Assessment'. This tool has gained great popularity due
446 to the wide application of 'The FICA Spiritual History Tool'—the basic version,
447 designed to assess the patient's spirituality. FICA for Self-Assessment contains four
448 groups of simple questions related to the four dimensions of spirituality. The first
449 group of questions concerns determining those beliefs that help in coping with stress
450 and give meaning to life. Second, determining how much these beliefs are important
451 in the process of making important life decisions. Another group of questions relate
452 to the need to belong to a community and to feel satisfied with this belonging. In
453 turn, the last group of questions concerns the need to make changes regarding spiri-
454 tual practices, talks with a representative of a religious/spiritual group [2].

455 **FICA for self-assessment**   t2.1

F—Faith and Belief	Do I have a spiritual belief that helps me cope with stress? With illness? What gives my life meaning?	t2.2 t2.3
I—Importance	Is this belief important to me? Does it influence how I think about my health and illness? Does it influence my healthcare decisions?	t2.4 t2.5
C—Community	Do I belong to a spiritual community (church, temple, mosque or another group)? Am I happy there? Do I need to do more with the community? Do I need to search for another community? If I don't have a community, would it help me if I found one?	t2.6 t2.7 t2.8 t2.9
A—Address in care	What should be my action plan? What changes do I need to make? Are there spiritual practices I want to develop? Would it help for me to see a chaplain, spiritual director, or pastoral counsellor?	t2.10 t2.11 t2.12

456
457 The George Washington Institute for Spirituality and Health [2]   t2.13

Another interesting tool is the tool developed by the Seattle Cancer Care Alliance. 458
As with the FICA, a list of open questions also appears in that tool. However, in the 459
case of 'Spiritual self-assessment', there are many more questions, and they refer 460
not to four but to nine dimensions of spirituality. The emerging questions concern, 461
among other support given by a religious community and special religious or spiri- 462
tual needs. Interesting are also questions regarding memories and spiritual / reli- 463
gious autobiography, beliefs about the meaning, healing and dying issues [29]. It is 464
also worth mentioning another tool developed as part of the Chaplain's On Hand 465
program by the Health Care Chaplaincy Network. The tool available online, unlike 466
the two above, is a list of questions with ready-made answers. The survey question- 467
naire contains eight items regarding, among others, care of himself, the image of 468
God/Higher Power and the most significant relationships [30]. The tools listed and 469
presented above are only selected examples of instruments available to spiritual 470
self-assess. It is difficult to find tools dedicated especially to nurses/midwives; how- 471
ever, those tools that are currently available seem to be also very useful for these 472
professional groups. Possibility of self-assessment of one's spiritual history and 473
insight into one's own spirituality may help to establish an open and trusting rela- 474
tionship with the patient. Frequent insight into one's own spirituality can facilitate 475
conversation about the patient's/client's spirituality. Assessing your own spiritual 476
history results not only in proficiency in asking appropriate questions and determin- 477
ing those dimensions of spirituality that may be particularly important for the 478
patient. Knowledge of your own spiritual history, awareness of how specific values 479
can be important for our lives, is also an opportunity to deeply understand the spiri- 480
tual history of the other person. Thanks to this, despite the difference of beliefs, it is 481
possible to establish nurse / midwife – patient relationship based on mutual respect 482
and deep trust. 483

Reflection
   – Describe your own actual intra-spiritual state according to the themes/
questions of the FICA for Self-Assessment tool. Did you find out anything
new about yourself and your own spirituality?
   – Share the outcomes with other students in a trustful context. Ask for
clarification to each other.
   – Discuss with each other what and how these intra-spiritual states
might affect the relationship with your patients/clients in general and more
specific for the spiritual care you are going to deliver in advance.
   – Turn back to the images at the top of this chapter. Reflect on them by
taking in account what you have learned from this chapter. What elements
from this chapter are useful in handling intrapersonal spirituality in such
situations?

References

1. EPICC. Spiritual Care Education Standard. www.epicc-network-org 2019. Last date visited 11-03-2021.
2. GWU. The George Washington Institute for Spirituality and Health. FICA for self-assessment. 2019. https://smhs.gwu.edu/gwish/clinical/fica/spiritual-history-tool. Accessed 9 Dec 2019.
3. Dossey BM, Keegan L. Holistic nursing: a handbook for practice. Ontario-London: Jones and Bartlett Publisher; 2009.
4. Bush T, Bruni N. Spiritual care as a dimension of holistic care: a relational interpretation. Int J Palliat Nurs. 2008;14(11):539–45.
5. Chirico F. Spiritual well-being in the 21st century: it is time to review the current WHO's health definition. J Health Social Sci. 2016;1(1):11–6.
6. Pert CB. Molecules of emotion—why you feel the way you feel. New York: Simon and Schuster; 1999.
7. Nolan S, Salthmarsh P, Leget C. Spiritual care in palliative care: working toward an EAPC task force. Eur J Palliat Care. 2011;18(2):86–9.
8. Haugan G. Life satisfaction in cognitively intact long-term nursing-home patients: symptom distress, well-being and nurse-patient interaction. In: Sarracino F, Mikucka M, editors. Beyond money—the social roots of health and well-being, chapter 10. New York: Nova Science; 2014. p. 165–211. ISBN: 978-1-63321-002.
9. Haugan G, Eide WM, André B, Wu Xi V, Rinnan E, Taasen SE, Kuven BM, Drageset J. Joy-of-life in cognitively intact nursing home patients: the impact of the nurse-patient interaction. Scand J Caring Sci. 2020;35(1):208–21. https://doi.org/10.1111/SCS.12836.
10. Haugan G, Moksnes UK, Løhre A. Intra-personal self-transcendence, meaning-in-life and nurse-patient interaction: powerful assets for quality of life in cognitively intact nursing home patients. Scand J Caring Sci. 2016;30(4):790–801.
11. Mongelluzzo NB. Understanding loss and grief. A guide through life changing events. Plymouth, Rowman & Littlefield. 2013.
12. Miller PA, Platter C. Plato's apology of Socrates: a commentary. Norman: University of Oklahoma; 2010.
13. Lévinas E. Totality and infinity: an essay on exteriority. Duquesne studies philosophical series, vol. 24. Pittsburgh, PA: Duquesne University Press; 1969. p. 307.
14. Lévinas E. Existence and existents. Pittsburgh, PA: Duquesne University Press; 1978. p. 113.
15. Lévinas E, Cohen T. Ethics and infinity: conversations with Philippe nemo 1982. Pittsburgh, PA: Duquesne University Press; 1985.
16. Eriksson K. The theory of caritative caring: A vision. Nursing Science Quarterly, 2007;20(3):201–202.
17. Rogers M. Utilising availability and vulnerability to operational spirituality. In: Béres L, editor. Practising spirituality. London: Palgrave; 2017. p. 144–62.
18. Levina E, Cohen T. Ethics and infinity: Conversations with Philippe Nemo 1982. Pittsburgh, Pennsylvania: Duquesne University Press. 1985.
19. Roxberg A, Eriksson K, Rehnsfeldt A, Fridlund B. The meaning of consolation as experienced by nurses in home-care setting. Journal of Clinical Nursing 2008;17:1079–87.
20. Thorne B. Person-centered counselling in action. 4th ed. London: SAGE; 2013.
21. Rogers M, Béres L. How two practitioners conceptualise spiritually competent practice. In: Wattis J, Curran S, Rogers M, editors. Spiritually competent practice in health care. Boca Raton: CRC; 2017. p. 53–70.
22. Rogers M, Wattis J, Stephenson J, Khan W, Curran S. A questionnaire-based study of attitudes to spirituality in mental health practitioners and the relevance of the concept of spiritually competent care. Int J Ment Health Nurs. 2019;28(5):1162–72. https://doi.org/10.1111/inm.12628.
23. Northumbria Community. Our rule of life. 2019. https://www.northumbriacommunity.org/. Accessed 1 Nov 2019.

24. Thorup CB, Rundqvist E, Roberts C, et al. Care as a matter of courage: vulnerability, suffer-   535
ing and ethical formation in nursing care. Scand J Caring Sci. 2012;26(3):427–35. https://doi.   536
org/10.1111/j.1471-6712.2011.00944.x.   537
25. Alsvag H. Martinsen K. Philosophy of caring. In: Alligood MR (ed.) Nursing theorists and   538
their work. 8th Edition. 2014; p. 147–70. Elsevier, St. Louis, MI.   539
26. Rankin E. & Delashmutt M.B. Finding spirituality and nursng presence: the students' chal-   540
lenge. Journal of Holistic Nursing. 2006;24(4)282–88.   541
27. Brown B. The gifts of imperfection: let go of who you think you're supposed to be embrace   542
who you are. Center City, MN: Hazelden; 2010.   543
28. Żołnierz J. Opieka duchowa w praktyce. Narzędzia do oceny duchowości pacjenta: FICA,   544
FACT. In: Chodźko E, Szymczyk P, editors. Wybrane prace z obszaru prawa, ekonomii i nauk   545
społecznych. Lublin: Wydawnictwo Naukowe TYGIEL; 2018. p. 223–32.   546
29. Seattle Cancer Care Alliance. Spiritual self-assessment. 2019. https://www.seattlecca.org/   547
emotional-and-spiritual-support/medical-support-services/spiritual-care-and-chaplaincy/sefl-   548
assessment. Accessed 9 Dec 2019.   549
30. Healthcare Chaplaincy Network. Spiritual self-assessment. 2019. http://chaplainsonhand.org/   550
cms/resources/tools-checklists/23-spiritual-self-assessment.html. Accessed 9 Dec 2019.   551

Suggested Reading   552

Janice C. Spiritual care in everyday nursing practice: a new approach. London: MacMillan   553
Education; 2013.   554
Koenig HG. Spirituality in patient care: why, how, when, and what. 3rd, Revised and Expanded ed.   555
Philadelphia, PA: Templeton Press; 2013.   556
Reed PG, Haugan G. Self-transcendence—a salutogenic process for well-being. Chapter 9. In: 557
Haugan G, Eriksson M, editors. Health promotion in health care—vital theories and research.   558
Berlin: Springer; 2020.   559

Chapter 6
Competence 2: Interpersonal Spirituality

Josephine Attard, Mohd Arif Atarhim, Beata Dobrowolska, Julie Jomeen, Joanne Pike, and Jacqueline Whelan

> **Learning Objectives**
> This chapter will enable you to:
>
> 1. Recognise the impact of the spiritual and cultural worldviews, beliefs and practices in the provision of care.
> 2. Develop the importance of effective reciprocal communication between nurses/midwives and patients which evoke feelings of companionship and compassionate care.
> 3. Promote the importance of spiritual care attitudes, such as sharing, caring, empathy, listening, touch and presence when delivering care.

J. Attard (✉)
University of Malta, Msida, Malta
e-mail: josephine.attard@um.edu.mt

M. A. Atarhim
The National University of Malaysia, Kuala Lumpur, Malaysia
e-mail: arifatarhim@ukm.edu.my

B. Dobrowolska
Medical University of Lublin, Lublin, Poland

J. Jomeen
School of Health and Human Sciences, Southern Cross University, Lismore, NSW, Australia
e-mail: julie.jomeen@scu.edu.au

J. Pike
Wrexham Glyndwr University, Wrexham, Wales, UK
e-mail: j.pike@glyndwr.ac.uk

J. Whelan
School of Nursing and Midwifery, Trinity College Dublin,
The University of Dublin,
Dublin, Ireland
e-mail: whelanj1@tcd.ie

6.1   Introduction

This chapter aims to address the three learning objectives outlined above and to support readers to develop their knowledge skills and attitudes in relation to interpersonal spirituality. We discuss why interpersonal spirituality is central to delivery
holistic care whist acknowledging their unique spiritual and cultural worldviews,
beliefs and practices. Through a combination of practice-based scenarios and reflective exercises, the reader will understand the key elements outlined in Competence
2 (Box 6.1) within the EPICC Spiritual Care Education Standard [1].

Box 6.1: Competence 2: Interpersonal Spirituality

Engages with persons' spirituality, acknowledging their unique spiritual and cultural worldviews, beliefs and practices		
Knowledge (cognitive)	Skills (functional)	Attitudes (behavioural)
– Understands the ways that persons express their spirituality. – Is aware of the different world/religious views and how these may impact upon persons' responses to key life events	– Recognises the uniqueness of persons' spirituality – Interacts with and responds sensitively to the person's spirituality	– Is trustworthy, approachable and respectful of persons' expressions of spirituality and different world/religious views

---

Interpersonal spirituality requires that nurses/midwives reflect on their individual attitudes and their relative impact on an ability to provide competent and effective spiritual care. Such personal reflection facilitates changes, where necessary, to
an individual practice whilst equally taking account of systemic barriers and facilitators to the provision of competent quality spiritual care. This chapter aims to
empower readers to reflect on the relevant knowledge, skills and attitudes relevant
to interpersonal spirituality to enable changes at an individual level. Also, to consider their role in influencing patients, clients, families and the wider organisation
within which they work. This chapter will address all three learning objectives in
turn by utilising the best available evidence in the field, providing critique and considering the application of the evidence that clarifies theory for practice.

6.2   Spiritual and Cultural Worldviews, Beliefs and Practices in the Provision of Care

Within increasingly diverse societies, brought about by migration and asylum seeking, spiritual, religious and cultural beliefs and practices can be unfamiliar and con-
fusing, thus presenting challenges for healthcare professionals. The Pew Research

Centre report [2] showed that there are eight categories of religions and beliefs 29
divided by rankings of population numbers, namely Christianity, Islam, Judaism, 30
Unaffiliated, Hinduism, Buddhism, Folk religion and Others. 31

Diversity in beliefs and worldviews can influence the understanding of spiritual- 32
ity and cultural views of the world. There are various opinions regarding the concept 33
of religion and spirituality. For some, religion and spirituality are closely related 34
whilst others consider that they are not necessarily interdependent [3]. This diver- 35
sity in views creates a challenge in nursing/midwifery to provide spiritual care that 36
meets the person's need, and it is argued that this requires understanding of an indi- 37
vidual's worldview to provide effective and individualised spiritual care. 38

Religion is a socio-cultural system that shapes behaviour, practices, morals and 39
ethics, worldviews, prophecies, sanctuaries and organisations. All of these elements 40
connect a human being with the supernatural, transcendental or spiritual [4]. For an 41
individual who adheres to religious beliefs, the life they lead from birth to the end 42
of life is very closely related to their faith, which provides strong and coherent 43
sources of meaning in life [5]. Similarly, in life-changing events such as birth or 44
illness, spirituality plays a vital role in finding meaning and purpose. Even for those 45
who do not follow a religion, for example those who do not believe in the existence 46
of God (atheist) or hold on to the unknowing existence of God (agnostic), their 47
beliefs still influence their worldview of health and illness [6]. 48

Levin's model [7] suggests a salutogenic effect of faith through five mechanisms 49
which includes: behavioural/conative, interpersonal, cognitive, affective and 50
psychophysiological. 51

Behavioural/conative emphasises the role of religion on health-promoting behav- 52
iour or motivation to be healthy. For example, many traditions of faith do not 53
encourage alcohol consumption, such as Islam. There are clear health benefits to 54
non-consumption, as well as social benefits in terms of antisocial or abusive behav- 55
iours. Other dietary and fasting behaviours also appear to have positive health 56
impacts [8]. 57

Interpersonal refers to the relationship between individuals who have similar 58
belief systems or with the higher-supreme being (or the unseen world). This interper- 59
sonal relationship can provide companionship and social support for the well-being 60
of the individual. For individuals who participate in their spiritual community either 61
formally or informally, this can establish friendships, which can reduce social isola- 62
tion resulting in positive concomitant which impacts on spiritual and mental health [8]. 63

Cognitive involves the thinking system of the individual in meaning-making and 64
sense-making of the world. For example, religion explains creation and what will 65
happen to this world. There are faith traditions that believe that there will be a 66
judgement day and an after-life. This helps to motivate the believer in present life, 67
to live well and prepare themselves for end of life peacefully. 68

Affective relates to the role of spiritual beliefs and practices in comfort, which in 69
turn impacts psychologically as a mediator for stress, with physiological benefits 70
such as improving the immune system [8]. 71

Psychophysiological refers to how faith promotes hope and optimism, which can 72
influence somatic responses. For example, by knowing that God will always help 73

74   during the illness trajectory will help to ease one's burden and capacity to endure
75   suffering.
76   This model illustrates the significant impact of faith on a person's health. It can
77   affect a person's coping mechanism, decision-making, social support, compliance
78   to treatment, use of complementary health approaches and general wellness [9].
79   It is of value to reflect further on how religious beliefs affect a person's coping
80   during illness. Religious coping mechanisms can be positive or negative. The posi-
81   tive effect involves secure attachment to God, a sense of belongingness with the
82   divine and faith community and the benefits of that as articulated above. Conversely,
83   the negative effect concerns feelings of abandonment and punishment from God,
84   often linked with avoidance of the faith community, and doubt in God's power [8].
85   It is therefore critical to acknowledge and to understand that an individual's religion
86   may manifest itself differently in times of personal crisis. Religious conflict or
87   struggle may not be conducive to recovery and well-being [8]; therefore, care must
88   be sensitive, seeking to respect the spiritual needs of the person, yet understand it in
89   the context of the illness experience, which requires observation and effective
90   communication.
91   It is also important to recognise that religious belief is not a necessary compo-
92   nent of spirituality, and that for some, religious and spiritual beliefs do not feature.
93   In such cases, support must be sought or provided that can provide meaning and
94   purpose to the person [9]. The middle-ranged theory of spiritual well-being in ill-
95   ness by O'Brien [10] suggests that each individual has the ability to seek spiritual
96   meaning in the experience of illness and that the search for spiritual meaning even-
97   tually leads to spiritual well-being. However, this requires open discussion and
98   acceptance of individual differences, which may not accord with our own personal
99   views and perspectives.
100   It is impossible in this chapter to discuss all faiths. A focus on some prevalent
101 world faiths, however, provides insight into how beliefs might impact on the provi-
102 sion of spiritual care. So, for example, whilst the focus on healthy living is relatively
103 consistent, it is underpinned by differing beliefs and philosophies, and some under-
104 standing of this facilitates more effective caring relationships.
105   Christians view the body as the temple of God, believing that a healthy lifestyle
106 can help the person to connect with the divine more fully. Muslims believe that the
107 body is entrusted from God and needs to be cared for. Thus, equilibrium in life and
108 choosing to do good rather than evil is important to achieve health. Jews perceive
109 their body as God's property; thus, the body needs to be taken care of and respected.
110 Hindus pursue health by balancing mind, body and soul with consciousness. The
111 *law of karma* (action and deed will reflect the positive or negative impact in this life
112 or the next life) plays a role in determining health. Buddhists believe that all things
113 are temporary and the existence in this world is not inherent or eternal [6]. In order
114 to provide spiritual care that can maximise the person's well-being and healing dur-
115 ing illness, therefore, it is vital to consider the person's worldview of health.
116   Another example of how different faiths view something as fundamental as diet
117 may also be helpful to consider. Diet for some faiths is about more than just fulfill-
118 ing a physical need. A case in point—although not universally the case—pertains to

Muslims, where both pork and alcohol are forbidden, and other meat must be   119
slaughtered according to Islamic Laws. If neither of these assumptions is guaran-   120
teed, seafood and vegetarian meals are only sufficient. Muslims will fast for   121
Ramadhan (Muslim calendar); however, exemption will be granted to those who are   122
ill and unable to perform the practice. Judaism also has some restrictions in diet   123
such as Kosher food, where meat has been prepared according to Jewish Law.   124
Shellfish, pork, rabbit and derivatives are strictly prohibited, and milk and meat   125
products are not eaten together [9]. Having knowledge of these practices is funda-   126
mentally linked, not only to good nutrition, but also to spiritual health.   127

Death is inevitable, yet faiths have different views on death. Understanding and   128
respecting these views is a critical part of care planning. Good spiritual care at the   129
time of death can facilitate a peaceful death, where individuals are assured that   130
practices according to their faith tradition will be observed [11].   131

Case Scenario

A woman had conceived a much wanted, eighth child, whilst visiting Mecca to pray for a last chance at motherhood. This conception was a 'blessing from Allah'. During a routine ultrasound scan, it was revealed to this woman that her unborn child has congenital heart problems. The effect of this news upon this woman was devastating, and she felt that the health service and God had failed her. The child was born with a severe heart defect and transferred to intensive care. The mother did not want to visit or learn of the child's problem. All she asked was whether a child with this condition had ever lived.

1. What are the spiritual needs of this client?
2. What do nurses and midwives need to know, be able to do, or think, in order to meet this client's needs?

Reflection:

How did this scenario make you feel? Reflect on those feelings and how you would manage them in a care encounter.

6.3 Effective, Verbal and Non-verbal Interaction between   132
Persons and Carers   133

The establishment of effective, reciprocal, person-centred communication is a pre-   134
requisite for compassionate spiritual care provision [12]. Interpersonal interaction is   135
innately relational. It firstly seeks to establish common ground that confirms the   136
individuality of the carer as a person and giver of care. Secondly, it respects the   137
humanity and diverse needs of the person receiving care [13].   138

Health professionals are uniquely placed to engage and respond to patients'   139
spiritual needs given the amount of direct contact time on a daily basis. It is   140
worth noting that the subjective nature of communication often requires   141

142 adaptation, renegotiation and acceptance as the patient moves through illness.
143 Some requesting dialogue about what spirituality means to help them cope or to
144 reconcile eventual death [8].
145   There is a definitive need to develop self-awareness as a lens for exploring, ques-
146 tioning and supporting patient perspectives and behavioural interactions. Research
147 has demonstrated that the professional's approach and manner determine the con-
148 textual parameters, quality of patient engagement and care outcomes [14]. This rec-
149 ognises the importance of increasing awareness and expanding sensitivities that
150 culminate in an increased sense of personal spirituality, in order to shape patient's
151 behaviours, actions, feelings and expressions of spirituality during interactions [14].
152   Research further suggests there is a need for health professionals to develop their
153 'spiritual literacy' [15]. This is an attempt to understand patients' diverse perspec-
154 tives and concerns; to develop a readiness to move beyond their comfort zone; to
155 foster trustworthiness and privacy and to champion an openness to act as a compan-
156 ion on the patient's journey that is reflective of the patient's healing process [15].
157 Such 'balancing of the self' demands getting to know strengths, limitations, bound-
158 aries and weaknesses in addition to handling beliefs [15]. Effective and reciprocal
159 verbal and non-verbal interactions are instrumental in supporting carers to develop
160 awareness. This involves recognising and delineating perceptions of feelings, per-
161 sonal preferences, priorities and innermost fears and concerns.

6.3.1   Therapeutic Interactions

163 Therapeutic interactions are viewed as dynamic mutual transactional processes.
164 This recognises the uniqueness of persons through awareness of the therapeutic use
165 of self and relationship trust-building, using verbal and non-verbal means to develop
166 caring and empathic practice [15, 16].
167   The purpose of a therapeutic interaction is to act as a primary means of support
168 by influencing participation in the patient, encouraging well-being and healing, sat-
169 isfaction and safe quality healthcare outcomes [16]. The significance of effective
170 interactions seeks to protect the patient's dignity, empowering them to tell their
171 story, to address individual concerns to discern and reconcile.
172   How the healthcare professional enters a person's world to form a therapeutic
173 relationship matters, as it provides support that recognises the integrity of the per-
174 son. Holding a broad view of spirituality and spiritual care is recognised as funda-
175 mental in understanding a person's spiritual and cultural worldviews, beliefs and
176 practices, thus finding common ground to ascertain a person's responses and impact
177 on key life events [12].
178   As discussed above, the nurse/midwife needs to find ways to acknowledge a
179 patient's unique worldviews to respect a patient's identity and express preferences
180 in all encounters. This promotes meaningful engagement to understand the person's

perspective of ill health or a new life changing experience. This demands that they   181
increase their sensitivity of their personal sense of spiritual awareness in order to   182
understand the everyday reality of the patient's experience [17].   183

6.3.2   Verbal and Non-verbal Interactions   184

Verbal and non-verbal messages are conveyed and linked to nurses' and midwives'   185
attitudes, life perspective, value sets, conscious use of self and personal views about   186
spirituality [15]. Personal warmth helps to forge a non-verbal connection between   187
the healthcare professional and the person, making the carer accessible with the   188
intent of listening attentively to fully engage with a patient's story. Compassion as   189
an extension of warmth and is directed towards being vulnerable, open and sensi-   190
tised to a patient's suffering in a non-judgemental manner, motivating the profes-   191
sional to listen to the person and alleviate it. Research proposes that carers who are   192
interested, caring and emotionally attuned to respond to patient perspectives attain   193
a healthy secure emotional bond with patients [18].   194

Verbal and non-verbal interactions represent broad integrative approaches that   195
are essential to each other in order to understand a person's health situation and   196
emotions, manage uncertainty and advance the self-care and level of involvement   197
the person to produce a healthy caring alliance [19]. Verbal communication relates   198
not only to the spoken word (7% of verbal message content) but to meaning gener-   199
ated from both verbal messages and non-verbal cues [20]. Pitch, tone and pattern   200
accounts for 38% of content that is all under the professional control for the pur-   201
poses of relaying thoughts and monitoring for changes in expressed emotions when   202
providing information and answering questions [20]. Professionals need to ascer-   203
tain a person's primary style of communicating to fit the person's situation given   204
that persons function most effectively within this [12]. This adaptation allows for   205
shared meanings to be socially constructed and interpreted.   206

The importance of effective verbal interaction strategies are highlighted in the   207
literature through a series of *micro-skills* [17]. The need to develop rapport by   208
adopting an appropriate sitting posture and getting to know the person through trust-   209
ful relations is significant as this develops a caring connection that allows the person   210
to be valued, accepted, supported and understood [17]. Making appropriate eye con-   211
tact, whilst listening actively, transmits a positive message and level of attention that   212
is indicative of empathy and interest. The need to ask questions (to develop open-   213
ness and clarification) is required for the purposes of eliciting a patients' situation,   214
distress, assessment, referral and feedback to clarify concerns and minimise misun-   215
derstandings. Ross and McSherry [21] have developed a model that uses two,   216
person-centred and open questions that encourage consideration of desires and   217
stresses, along with what matters to them without being overburdened, thus provid-   218
ing an opportunity to reflect and respond upon feelings.   219

6.3.3   What Is Most Important to You Now? How Can We Help?

The need to attune to a person's feelings, particularly in the presence of distress, is important to ascertain the 'type' and 'intensity' of inner feelings [22] and to gain insights [21]. Seven diverse universal emotions exist across cultures to gain insights, specifically anger, fear, sadness, disgust, surprise, contempt and happiness [21]. Other practical strategies highlighted in the literature for thinking and reflecting on feelings and identifying a person's concerns include silence, storytelling, metaphors and rituals.

Non-verbal communication is viewed as communication without the presence of speech, which is directed towards transmitting attitudes and feelings about ourselves and others [22]. Multiple effective modes of non-verbal communication exist which can occur simultaneously through interactions, posture, proximity, touch, body movements, facial expression, eye behaviour, vocal cues, use of time, physical presence and environmental cues [22]. How the nurse/midwife moves within an intimate space has the capacity to positively or negatively impact boundaries, relationships, along with receiving and providing information. Lack of awareness of safe distances has the propensity to violate a person's proximal space. It is important for the professional to negotiate a process of informed consent so as not to threaten or compromise truths within the nurse/midwife relationship with the patient.

Non-verbal communication needs to be used consciously, to accurately interpret patient's feelings. Although research has demonstrated that non-verbal interactions 'speak loudest' and 'cancel out' verbal messages when incongruence exists between the two, there still remains a need to qualify such perceptions by verbal means [22].

Individuals perceive how they are accepted through a health professional's listening responses and interest. Active listening is an intentional observational activity that is developed with, time [14]. This culminates in a facilitative response for the carer to hear and listen to the patient's story to ascertain primary feelings and conversational themes that shape a person's values, identity and experience of illness through non-verbal means [18]. How patients feel can be ascertained through seven indicators: feelings, words, emotion in the voice, emotion expressed in the face or body, protesting too much, self-contraindications, which indicate inner conflict, discussion of parental or other crucial needs, satisfying relationship and recognising negative feelings [14]. Touch constitutes a powerful listening response to make patients feel comfortable and secure. Fundamentally, the importance of listening is for the carer to be present and attentive. This helps to make sense of what is heard, in order to know, how to respond to expressed patient needs or concerns to minimise any misunderstanding.

Nursing and midwifery education is mandated to promote interpersonal approaches to spiritual care by orientating the student towards compassion. This needs the development of a safe space; an inclusive approach to care underpinned by self-awareness; holding a broad worldview; developing an increased sense of personal spirituality; along with sensitive discerning interactions that are timed, paced, validated and adapted to fit the patient's situation [17].

6.4   Evoking Companionship and Compassionate Care

As discussed above, the essence of nursing/midwifery work can be described by its relational character. As professionals, we are aware that our work is never done just for work itself but always for other people and in relation to other people. Providing holistic nursing/midwifery care, in each of its permeating dimensions, requires the ability to establish, develop and maintain genuine relationships with patients/client/family members, and also with people with whom they cooperate in multidisciplinary therapeutic teams.

Spiritual care is particularly relational in nature. It touches the inner self, is personal and thus a very intimate human interaction, and as such is only possible in a one-to-one, personal relationship. Practitioners need a patient's consent to be 'let into' their world in order to recognise and assess spiritual needs and provide effective care. For this reason, *trust* is recognised as important attribute of spiritual nursing care [22]. In trustful relationship, the patient feels they are treated with respect and their value as a person is acknowledged. Only then, through genuinely 'being with' the patient in the process of their care, treatment and recovery, can spiritual needs be identified and met.

The Spiritual Care Education Standard for undergraduate nursing/midwifery students [1] indicates the necessary attitudinal attributes for spiritual care competency development. Specifically, being 'open and respectful to persons' diverse expressions of spirituality' in intrapersonal spirituality; along with being 'trustworthy, approachable and respectful of persons' expressions of spirituality…' in interpersonal spirituality; and being 'open, approachable and non-judgmental' when assessing and planning spiritual care. These help to facilitate the behaviours outlined above as necessary.

Connectedness with patients in an open and trustful relationship makes space for compassion, which has been identified as a core element of nursing practice and the heart of nursing/midwifery care (compassionate care). Specifically, it is impossible to practice spiritual nursing care without compassion. Compassion is an 'active feeling', which means that there is an obligation to act in order to make a change in a patient's situation as much as it is possible and within the scope of competence. There are evident positive impacts of practising compassion on patients' health outcomes and recovery, the quality of care provided, as well as satisfaction with their work [16].

In their review on compassion in nursing practice and education, Younas and Maddigan [16] identified three direct indicators of compassionate care, i.e., recognising, accepting and alleviating patients' suffering. They also proposed four foundational elements of practising compassion:

1. Authentic presence (connecting meaningfully with patients, being present and building genuine relationship with them, doing and sharing with one another and being in solidarity with patients).
2. Empathy and understanding (as described previously).
3. Respect (respecting patients' values, choices, autonomy and dignity to make them comfortable to share their happiness and suffering, involving patients in decision-making processes, being kind and communicating with them in a kind manner, remembering what patients had shared with us, and spending time with patients).
4. Openness to patients' needs (trying to understand, respect and carefully meet patients' needs, recognising patients' concerns and emotions).

Being aware of the attributes of compassion facilitates an increased knowledge about how to practice compassionate care, and how education should be delivered to make compassionate care real in clinical settings [16]. Effective student reflection on their personal spirituality and the spirituality of others can be an appropriate teaching and learning strategy to promote knowledge and application of compassionate care. This can take a variety of methods, for example: class discussion, role-plays, use of stories (based on real experiences of health care) reflecting on personal experience of being a family member of a patient, role models (given by teachers, mentors and also peers) [23]. A wide range of scenarios for the development of nursing/midwifery students' competencies to provide compassionate spiritual care can be found in the EPICC Adoption Toolkit [24].

To understand the meaning of compassion in nursing/midwifery care, having personal experience of receiving compassionate care, as well as practice of self-compassion, is important [23]. States of vulnerability enable us to discover how meaningful assistance, the presence of other people and the criticality of support can be. It is also fundamental experience to build into nursing/midwifery education. In the case of spiritual care, reflection on personal vulnerability can support practitioners to identify their own limits and strengths in the process of recognising their own spirituality and the spirituality of their patients [23]. The process involves sensitive and delicate issues and requires practitioners to be ready to deal with their own emotions as well as emotions of patients and/or their family members. The Spiritual Care Education Standard [1] identifies a 'willingness to deal with emotions' as an attitude critical to achieving competency in providing spiritual care.

Working with emotions may be challenging, especially for younger student nurses/midwives, who may find it difficult to establish deep and close connectedness with patient whose life experiences they cannot echo. To develop and maintain respectful connectedness with patient/family members and provide compassionate spiritual care requires time. Sharing time with patients is difficult in contemporary healthcare systems which face staff shortage, and thus, nurses complain about lack

of time even for very basic nursing procedures. In such circumstances, the role of   345
nursing managers is critical to work on strategies that potentially release time for a   346
holistic approach to patient/family members in their institution.   347

This is also important when planning and organising clinical training for under-   348
graduate nursing/midwifery students. The teaching–learning environment in place-   349
ment should make it possible to understand the meaning of holistic nursing care   350
(with spiritual care as a vital part) and methods of its implementation in daily prac-   351
tice [21]. Therefore, placements and mentorship need to be conducive to supporting   352
students to learn how to make time to establish and develop a close relationship with   353
patient/family members and provide compassionate care.   354

6.5   Promoting Spiritual Care Attitudes   355

The caring professions have long claimed a holistic viewpoint of the patient, in   356
other words, viewing the patient not as though they are separate components of   357
body, mind and spirit, but that these are indivisible from one another and therefore   358
one. A continuous and harmonious interaction between the innermost core spirit,   359
the mind and the body, is required to maintain an individual's health. An approach   360
such as this is conceived as meaning that each of the concepts of mind, body and   361
spirit are a way of understanding certain manifestations of the whole person.   362

6.5.1   The Body and Its Centrality to Spiritual Care   363

Where the person is under stress, for example during a significant diagnosis or   364
where there is critical illness, spirituality has been said to come to the fore. This   365
means that the spiritual variable may affect the coping mechanisms of the person   366
who is under stress and may therefore be called upon in order to assist the person in   367
coping. If this is true, then nurses have an ethical imperative to assist the person to   368
utilise the spiritual aspect of their being in this way.   369

Pierre Bourdieu [25] endowed the body with symbolic value—a 'physical capi-   370
tal'—so maintenance of the body is important to people. Sociologically speaking,   371
Shilling [26] asserts that the body in life and in health is crucial to the person's sense   372
of self, and therefore, if broken, may cause the patient to suffer a loss of self, a con-   373
cern which may also impact on the person's spirituality. Caring for the body then   374
requires concern for the person's spirit, though this must be undertaken with caring   375
attention. Touch, as discussed above, is viewed as a therapeutic use of self and an   376
expression of spiritual care when practiced with intention and caring compassion.   377

6.5.2 Human Relationships, Listening and Attending

Whilst medicine may not have all the answers for a patient facing suffering, when that person is able to share their concerns with others, a restorative effect can often be seen. Russell [27] identified that when public services respond to people in a personalised way, feelings of worthiness ensue; people feel they are important and that their well-being matters to others. It follows that our spiritual lives are to do with relationships to those around us and in how it manifests in our lives as we share them with others.

6.5.3 Spirituality and Presence

Spirituality is a concept that is still developing in healthcare and identifying that presence and caring have a spiritual basis may confuse the picture further. Added to this concern is that professionals tend not to use language that conveys spirituality when describing spiritual care. Instead, they use words that are concerned with communication and that convey presence as they discuss listening or 'being there' for the patient. Therefore, it seems a sensible alternative to describe expressions of spiritual care, particularly as they have been developed and embedded in nursing culture over time.

Whilst is it related to concepts of caring such as empathy and support, 'presencing' is a way of being that requires that the practitioner give something of oneself and *fully recognises* the patient's suffering [28]. Transcendent presence occurs when a healthcare professional is present for a patient physically, mentally, emotionally and spiritually. 'Presencing' demands the practitioner to be fully present with the person, even when the situation cannot be altered [28]. It could be argued that such an intervention as this is the ultimate in caring, if spirituality is concerned with the person's whole being, and holistic care is the aim of caring practice. Spiritual care can thus be said to support the patient experiencing stress or anxiety at times of need by providing caring touch, listening and presence.

> **Reflective Exercise**
> This account is taken from a nurse's reflective diary.
> I was working as a bank nurse for a local nursing home and was doing the night shift. It was just me and an agency carer and it was mad busy. The carer didn't know the residents and I didn't know them well, but I knew the routine and we just got on with it together. I was doing the medicine round, and as usual, it seemed to take ages, going round to each resident's room with what they needed.

At handover at the beginning of the shift, I had been warned about one particular man who was 'always on the bell' ringing for assistance constantly, but 'when you get there, he doesn't want anything love', said the sister at handover. True to my handover, the bell was rung often, and each time I went, there was a little something that was needed, but each time I went, I was being pulled away from my duties for the other residents, and I was, to be honest, getting a bit frustrated.

I thought about what I could do, and then I said to him 'Mr. B, please can you give me a little while just to get the medicine round done then I can come and spend some time with you?' He agreed, but then rang the bell within 15 min. I tried again, with the same plea, adding, 'I should be done by about eleven, could I come back then, and we can have a chat and I'll bring you a drink and things?'

I was just about done, and it was just after 11 (he had rung twice again before then!) and I went back, smiling and saying 'See, I said I'd be back!' I said I had half an hour before I had to go and was that OK? He nodded. I did all the 'nursey' things, pillows, repositioning, giving him a drink, washing his hands and face and combing his hair and then I sat down beside him and asked him if he wanted to hold my hand. In answer, he held out his hand and looked at me. I looked back and said nothing but gave him my full attention. I was there for about 20 min, just sitting, and then, when I said, 'You OK?' he nodded and smiled a tiny bit and closed his eyes.

- Reflect on the above scenario and consider what did the nurse do in this scenario that illustrates both presence and expresses spiritual care?
- Would you feel confident to act in this way?

6.5.4   Holistic Meaningful Care

Patients are aware of the ways in which staff give holistic and meaningful care. Pike [29] identified how patients expressed their experience of spiritual care, using the language of communication, evidencing how they felt staff comforted them and connected with them in the 'everyday' interactions of the day case surgery unit. Being present with and connecting to another underpins spiritual care [29]. However, if healthcare professionals are not always aware of their therapeutic potential in the caring relationship, raising awareness of the potential for giving care spiritually by intentionally using a spiritual caring approach, along with listening to and connecting with the patient, will enhance their experience of care.

6.6   Summary of the Main Points for Learning

Nurses and midwives will inevitably see patients and clients with a wide variety of unique spiritual and cultural worldviews, religions, beliefs and practices. Education must reflect that diversity of views and opinions, requiring a broad universal approach to the teaching of spirituality, without overly generalising the concept; yet explaining the impact of spiritual and religious beliefs and practices in decisions that may affect care. It has been argued here that knowledge and skill development to underpin cultural competence will support nursing/midwifery students to engage in the provision of effective spiritual care.

Two models, the Actioning Spirituality and Spiritual Care Education and Training (ASSET), and the Assessment, Communication, Cultural Negotiation and Compromise, Empathy and Respect, Sensitivity and Security (ACCESS) models [30], guide spiritual care education and transcultural care practice in nursing and midwifery. However, for nurses and midwives to be culturally and spiritually competent, they must also learn to suspend their own cultural values and traditions and to reflect on any differences that may exist between their patients 'or clients' values and their own.

A reflective model for nurse education is proposed to enhance culturally responsive care, since critical reflection in clinical practice is identified as an important process to enhance spiritual practice. Consideration of how healthcare professionals acknowledge their own biases and enable safe expression through effective communication, compassion and therapeutic interaction is underpinned by empathy, listening, touch and presence. Collectively, this adds meaning to interpersonal relationships.

References

1. EPICC. Spiritual Care Education Standard. 2019a. https://blogs.staffs.ac.uk/epicc/files/2019/06/EPICC-Spiritual-Care-Education-Standard.pdf. Accessed 2 Dec 2019.
2. Hackett C, Grim BJ. The global religious landscape. Washington, DC: Pew Research Center Report; 2015.
3. Hill PC, Pargament KI, Hood RW, McCullough J, Swyers JP, Larson DB. Conceptualizing religion and spirituality: points of commonality, points of departure. J Theory Soc Behav. 2000;30:10021–8308.
4. Kaddourah B, Abu-Shaheen A, Al-Tannir M. Nurses' perceptions of spirituality and spiritual care at five tertiary care hospitals in Riyadh, Saudi Arabia: a cross-sectional study. Oman Med J. 2018;33(2):154–8.
5. Crescioni AW, Baumeister RF. The four needs for meaning, the value gap, and how (and whether) society can fill the void. In: The experience of meaning in life: classical perspectives, emerging themes, and controversies; 2013.
6. Taylor EJ. Religion: a clinical guide for nurses. Berlin: Springer; 2012.
7. Levin J. How faith heals: a theoretical model. Explore. 2009;5(2):77–96.
8. Taylor EJ. Health outcomes of religious and spiritual belief, behaviour, and belonging: implication for healthcare professionals. In: Timmins F, Caldeira S, editors. Spirituality in healthcare: perspectives for innovative practice. Cham: Springer; 2019. p. 67–82.
9. Rumun AJ. Influence of religious beliefs on healthcare practice. Int J Educ Res. 2014;2(4):1.
10. O'Brien ME. Spirituality in nursing: standing on holy ground. 6th ed. Burlington, MA: Jones & Bartlett Learning; 2018.

11. Taylor EJ, Park CG, Pfeiffer JB. Nurse religiosity and spiritiual care. Journal of advanced   460
    Nursing. 2014;70(11):2612–21.   461
12. Fleischer S, Berg A, Zimmermann M, Wuste K, Behrens J. Nurse patient interaction and com-   462
    munication; a systematic literature review. J Public Health. 2009;17:339–53.   463
13. Clarke J. Spiritual care in everyday nursing practice, a new approach. London: Palgrave   464
    Macmillan; 2013.   465
14. O'Hagan SM, Elder C, Pill J, Woodward-Kron R, McNamara T, Webb G, McColl G. What   466
    counts as effective communication in nursing? Evidence from nurse educators' and clinicians'   467
    feedback on nurse interactions with simulated patients. J Adv Nurs. 2014;2014(70):1344–56.   468
15. Giske T, Cone PH. Discerning the healing path- how nurses assist patient spirituality in diverse   469
    health care settings. J Clin Nurs. 2015;24:2926–35.   470
16. Younas A, Maddigan J. Proposing a policy framework for nursing education for fostering   471
    compassion in nursing students: a critical review. J Adv Nurs. 2019;75:1621–36.   472
17. Taylor Johnson E. Verbal responses to spiritual pain. In: What do I say? Talking with patients   473
    about spirituality. Philadelphia, PA: Templeton Press; 2007. p. 53–100.   474
18. Greenberg LS. Emotion in the therapeutic relationship in emotion focused therapy. In: Gilbert   475
    P, Leahy R, editors. The therapeutic relationship in the cognitive behavioural therapies. Hove: 476
    Routledge; 2007. p. 43–62.   477
19. Pinto RZ, Ferreira M, Oliveira V, Franco M, Adams R, Maher C. Patient centred commu-   478
    nication is associated with positive therapeutic alliance; a systematic review. J Physiother.   479
    2012;58:77–87.   480
20. McCabe C, Timmins F. Communication skills for nursing practice. London: Palgrave   481
    McMillan; 2013.   482
21. Ross L, McSherry W. Two questions that ensure person-centred spiri-   483
    tual care. Nurs Standard. 2018. https://rcni.com/nursing-standard/features/   484
    two-questions-ensure-person-centred-spiritual-care-137261.   485
22. Silverman J, Kurtz S, Draper J. Building the relationship. In: Skills for communicating with   486
    patients. London: Radcliffe Publishing; 2013. p. 112–44.   487
23. Giske T, Cone PH. Opening up to learning spiritual care of patients: a grounded theory study   488
    of nursing students. J Clin Nurs. 2012;21:2006–15.   489
24. EPICC. Adoption toolkit. 2019b. http://blogs.staffs.ac.uk/epicc/resources/epicc-adoption-   490
    toolkit/. Accessed 2 Dec 2019.   491
25. Bourdieu P. Outline of a theory of practice. Cambridge: Cambridge University Press; 1997.   492
26. Shilling C. The body and social theory. 2nd ed. Thousand Oaks, CA: Sage; 2003.   493
27. Russell J. New labour's great mistake is to think we are all automatons: the party's robot cal-   494
    culus ignored the fact that public services are about people's real, social and emotional needs,   495
    The Guardian. 2009; p. 27. http://www.guardian.cu.uk/commentisfree/2009/jul/14/targets-   496
    nhs-care-crime-bureaucracy. Accessed 11 Dec 2009.   497
28. Osterman P, Schwartz-Barcott D. Presence: four ways of being there. Nurs Forum.   498
    1996;31(2):23–30.   499
29. Pike J. Searching for the hidden: a phenomenological study exploring the spiritual aspects of   500
    impending day case surgery from patient and staff perspectives. Unpublished PhD. University   501
    of Wales. 2012.   502
30. Narayanasamy A. The impact of empirical studies of spirituality and culture on nurse educa-   503
    tion. J Clin Nurs. 2006;2006(15):840–51.   504

Suggested Reading   505

Jordon KD, Masters KS, Hooker SA, Ruiz JM, Smith TW. An interpersonal approach to religious-   506
    ness and spirituality: implications for health and well-being. J Personality. 2014;82(5):418–31.   507
Linhares CH. The lived experiences of midwives with spirituality in childbirth: Mana from heaven.   508
    J Midwif Women Health. 2012;57(2):165–71.   509
Pesut B. Developing spirituality in the curriculum: worldviews, intrapersonal connectedness, inter-   510
    personal connectedness. Nurs Educ Perspect. 2003;24(6):290–4.   511

Chapter 7
Competence 3: Spiritual Care, Assessment and Planning

Wilfred McSherry, Karnsunaphat Balthip, C. Swift, Olga Riklikienė, Sarah McKay, and Yanping Niu

W. McSherry (✉)
Department of Nursing, School of Health and Social Care, University Hospitals of North Midlands NHS Trust, Staffordshire University, Stoke-on-Trent, Staffordshire, England, UK

VID University College, Bergen/Oslo, Norway
e-mail: w.mcsherry@staffs.ac.uk

K. Balthip
Child and Adolescent Development Research Unit, Faculty of Nursing, Prince of Songkla University, Hat Yai, Songkhla, Thailand

C. Swift
Director of Chaplaincy and Spirituality, Methodist Homes (MHA) Derby, Derbyshire, England, UK

University of Staffordshire, Stoke-on-Trent, Staffordshire, England, UK
e-mail: chris.swift@mha.org.uk

O. Riklikienė
Department of Nursing and Care, Faculty of Nursing, Medical Academy, Lithuanian University of Health Sciences, Kaunas, Lithuania
e-mail: olga.riklikiene@lsmuni.lt

S. McKay
The Clatterbridge Cancer Centre, Liverpool, England, UK

Y. Niu
Department of Nursing, Changzhi Medical College, Shanxi, China

Learning Objectives
This chapter will enable you to:

1. Understand the nature of spiritual care and how one can assess and plan this within clinical practice.
2. Explain what is meant by the term spiritual assessment and the different approaches that this may involve.
3. Identify the requisite knowledge necessary to undertake a spiritual assessment and the associated values and skills to conduct this competently and confidently.

7.1   Introduction

In this chapter, we explore what is meant by spiritual care and explain how a spiritual assessment may be undertaken. We discuss why spiritual assessment is central to the planning and delivery of spiritual care by identifying the requisite knowledge, skills and attitudes necessary to do this confidently and competently. Through a combination of practice-based scenarios and reflective exercises, the reader will cover the key elements outlined in Competence 3 (Box 7.1) within the EPICC Spiritual Care Education Standard [1].

A great deal has been written about spiritual assessment, with the first real attempt to formalise this in nursing being developed by Ruth Stoll [2] in her article titled 'Guidelines for spiritual assessment'. These guidelines focus on four primary areas of a person's life: religious beliefs and practices, understanding of God or deity, sources of hope and strength and the relationships between spiritual beliefs and health. Stoll's pioneering work has been adapted and used within many different context, settings and professions. Because these guidelines were published in the United States, some aspects of them may be difficult to transfer into other

---

Box 7.1: Competence 3: Spiritual Care, Assessment and Planning

Assesses spiritual needs and resources using appropriate formal or informal approaches, and plans spiritual care, maintaining confidentiality and obtaining informed consent

Knowledge (cognitive)	Skills (functional)	Attitudes (behavioural)
– Understands the concept of spiritual care – Is aware of different approaches to spiritual assessment – Understands other professionals' roles in providing spiritual care	– Conducts and documents a spiritual assessment to identify spiritual needs and resources – Collaborates with other professionals – Be able to appropriately contain and deal with emotions	– Is open, approachable and non-judgemental – Has a willingness to deal with emotions

worldviews, cultures and life situations. Having stated this, the four primary areas   22
do provide valuable insights into what people globally consider fundamental to their   23
lives, such as beliefs, what provides meaning and purpose and where they may find   24
or seek support during key life events.   25

McSherry [3] in the absence of any authoritative definitions proposes spiritual   26
assessment is '…an attempt to enquire positively and unobtrusively with a patient/   27
client or their carers into areas of life that are associated with their health and well-   28
being. It is more than just an enquiry into physical health. It is an exploration of the   29
person's psychosocial and spiritual functioning'.   30

This definition implies that spiritual assessment must be undertaken sensitively,   31
respectfully, preserving the dignity of the individual. It suggests it must be part of a   32
holistic, person-centred approach and implies that spiritual assessment may take   33
many forms ranging from a simple screening to an in-depth spiritual history.   34

7.2 Theory, Rationale and Evidence Base for Spiritual Care   35

There are many reasons why effective assessment of spiritual needs is desirable and of   36
value. For example, it is hard to argue convincingly that care is person-centred if key   37
elements of personal significance are ignored. It has also become increasingly clear that   38
beliefs hold clinical value in the treatment of conditions and can be of benefit in the later   39
stages of life [4]. It follows that the identification and support of spiritual convictions   40
and practices have the potential to improve the well-being of people in receipt of care.   41

Evidence of intentional approaches to the organisation of religious care in hos-   42
pitals can be found at least as far back as the fourteenth century [5]. At that time,   43
the needs of patients were classified in relation to religious themes, with chaplains   44
organised to provide various sacraments in response. Until the twenty-first century,   45
spirituality was still widely employed as a variant way of speaking about religion.   46
However, with increasing social change, historic forms of religious identification   47
have become less pronounced for many populations. Whereas a person's religion   48
was once strongly connected with a stable sense of community and belonging, in   49
more recent years spirituality has become uncoupled from religion and developed   50
a life of its own. People may describe themselves as 'spiritual not religious', and   51
their spirituality may develop and change in significant ways. This fluidity and   52
dynamic character present certain challenges to public institutions, not least hospi-   53
tals, when it comes to offering spiritual support. This is especially true with regard   54
to recording spirituality and spiritual needs and allowing for the possibility that   55
these may evolve and change during a patient's journey. Effective assessment   56
therefore becomes a vital tool for high-quality care, in order to achieve accurate   57
and meaningful support. No longer can the allocation of a label, such as Muslim or   58
Sikh, be seen as an adequate piece of information for the purposes of spiritual care.   59

While there is a small amount of evidence that religious needs in the healthcare   60
population were diversifying in the twentieth century, it is only in the last 30 years   61
that most Western countries have experienced a widening range of multi-faith and   62
non-religious belief. In addition to demographic change, there has also been a shift   63
of perception and attitudes supported by equality legislation and active programmes   64

65   designed to foster a culture where difference and diversity are seen as desirable
66   characteristics.
67   It follows that the characteristics of assessment and planning for spiritual and
68   pastoral care should be shaped by the nature of need, be reflexive and adaptable and
69   be seen as a continuous process, rather than a one-off acquisition of stable data. It
70   should also be noted that spiritual needs assessment may, in itself, be a form of
71   pastoral care intervention. However, before we look at the different approaches to
72   spiritual assessment, we need to understand what is meant by spiritual care.

73   ## 7.2.1   Spiritual Care: Fact or Fiction?

> **Reflective Exercise 1**
> *What do you think about when you hear the word 'spiritual care'? Take a
> minute and write down your own definition of 'spiritual care'. What are some
> specific characteristics of good spiritual care? The purpose of the exercise is
> to encourage you to think about what spiritual care consists of. There are no
> right or wrong answers.*

74   Having reflected on your own definition of spiritual care, a useful starting point
75   might be to compare your definition with the one that is used in the EPICC Spiritual
76   Care Education Standard (2019, p. 2).

77   *Care which recognises and responds to the human spirit when faced with life-changing
78   events (such as birth, trauma, ill health, loss) or sadness, and can include the need for
79   meaning, for self-worth, to express oneself, for faith support, perhaps for rites or prayer or
80   sacrament, or simply for a sensitive listener. Spiritual care begins with encouraging human
81   contact in compassionate relationship and moves in whatever direction need requires.*

82   • *How does your definition compare, are there any similarities or difference?*
83   Reading through this definition, it is evident spiritual care is dynamic, needs led,
84   by that we mean it is the individual patient, person and women who express their
85   own spiritual needs. These needs may arise at key life events as described around
86   birth, trauma, illness or death. Spiritual care is not just about the negative aspects of
87   life it is also about celebrating events and occasions that bring joy and happiness.
88   From this definition, spiritual care is not about imposing a set of beliefs, value
89   behaviours or practices. It is about accompanying the person, coming alongside
90   them, being present, listening and supporting. It is not about making judgements, it
91   is enabling the person to be themselves and to express their own spiritual needs
92   whether these be religious practices, rituals or just finding time to be still and silent.
93   It is clear from this definition that providing spiritual care is in fact, an integral part
94   of nursing, midwifery and healthcare practice. It is not some fictitious or imaginary
95   concept; it is a fundamental and real dimension of all care. The challenge for all
96   nursing and midwifery practitioners is given the diversity of need that spiritual care
97   may encompass how do we undertake a spiritual assessment and how can we use the

outcomes of this assessment to plan nursing care that it is truly patient-centred, compassionate and holistic. In order to achieve this goal and level of competence, there is a specific knowledge base required around the delivery of spiritual care.

7.3   The Knowledge Base for Spiritual Care

This section considers the existing knowledge for spiritual care assessment and planning. It provides an overview of some of the commonly used approaches to spiritual assessment explaining the difference between screening and other more in-depth methods such as history taking.

In 2011 Monod et al. [6] identified 35 published measures of spirituality. All these measures related to spirituality and health in some form. While some instruments focused on the current spiritual well-being of patients, none addressed the specific concept of spiritual distress. The authors also noted the need for assessment to be effective in identifying a changing spiritual state over time.

One of the leading assessment tools is the Functional Assessment of Chronic Illness Therapy–Spiritual Well-Being Scale (FACIT-sp) [7]. A study by Vlasblom et al. [8] found that when used by nursing staff, the instrument led to more referrals to chaplaincy, but it was unclear whether this meant that nurses were therefore providing less spiritual care themselves. However, it should be noted that any serious attempt to assess spiritual needs may in effect be providing spiritual care within the process of assessment. Asking people serious questions about faith and belief in a compassionate way can increase the sense that these are recognised and affirmed as valuable in the patient's life.

Very often forms of assessment place an emphasis on meaning or meaning-making. There are questions concerning this when people demonstrate cognitive differences, which may arise from several causes including dementia. How meaning is expressed and identified must be a consideration in the assessment of spiritual need if we are to avoid an approach which may become narrow and exclusive.

Discourse analysis of a chaplain's interactions with patients in a UK hospital illustrates some of the peculiar dynamics of assessment and care. This research found that the chaplain used everyday language in a manner which was highly effective in eliciting narratives relevant to patient care and well-being. The researchers found that 'conversing openly and intimately about issues of faith and religion … without following a predetermined agenda is something that is artfully and strategically constructed' ([9], p. 57). In other words, exchanges which appeared normal and everyday were shaped in a way that elicited details of spiritual identity and need without appearing to be technical or reductionist.

Before going any further, it is important to clarify several terms associated with spiritual assessment, McSherry and Ross [10] in their work raised awareness of the different approaches to spiritual assessment and the potential challenges these presented. A summary of the main approaches to spiritual assessment outlined in are Box 7.2.

Box 7.2: Approaches to Spiritual Assessment

Direct methods	*This involves asking a direct question such as an enquiry about a person's personal religious or spiritual belief. This direct approach could also be considered a form of initial screening or enquiry*	t2.1 t2.2 t2.3
Indicator-based models	*These approaches follow a specific protocol or pathway such as those associated with spiritual distress or diagnosis*	t2.4 t2.5
Audit tools	*Many healthcare organisations actively seek to establish how well these areas are being addressed within practice by undertaking local audits*	t2.6 t2.7
Value clarification	*Scales used to explore perceptions and understandings of spirituality*	t2.8 t2.9
Indirect methods	*Cues observed in the environment that may indicate a spiritual need*	t2.10 t2.11
Acronym-based models	*Simple models or approaches often used within an initial assessment such as FICA (discussed below)*	t2.12 t2.13

Adapted from [3, 10, 11]   t2.14

Closer analysis of Box 7.2 suggests that some of these approaches may be formal and direct while others are less formal and indirect such as those methods using observation. One approach that is also used by some health and social care professional such as social workers and chaplains is taking a spiritual history.

7.3.1 Screening

In most cases the advantage of screening for spiritual needs lies in enabling large numbers of patients to be triaged without exceeding the tolerance of health staff to carry it out. Patient and user numbers can be vast, and healthcare staff have very limited time to spend on something which they may not feel is essential. It also provides structure for a conversation which can be reflective and about more than 'what religion are you?' Used well a tool like this can communicate a hint of what spiritual care is like (reflective); that it is not exclusively about religion and enables prompt referrals to a specialist, such as a chaplain, for a more detailed assessment.

7.3.2 History Taking

More often associated with the medical world, history taking can generate a much deeper and more comprehensive insight into someone's spiritual past. It enables both the person taking the history and the patient/user, to build a common understanding of the beliefs, associations and priorities of the person at the point they begin a course of treatment or support.

7.3.3 Formal Assessment   159

The work produced by the EPICC project establishes the need to assess 'spiritual   160
needs and resources using appropriate formal or informal approaches, and plans   161
spiritual care, maintaining confidentiality and obtaining informed consent'. It is tell-   162
ing and significant that emphasis falls on both needs and resources. It is recognised   163
widely that spiritual convictions and practices can aid someone during a period of   164
illness or adversity. Effective assessment is key to exploring the relationship of reli-   165
gion and spirituality to an episode or prolonged period of illness. While some ele-   166
ment of assessment, albeit informal in many cases, has featured in the work of   167
chaplains, there has been a lack of a formal framework for health professionals   168
more widely.   169

The EPICC work articulates the case for supporting spirituality in patients' lives,   170
not least because of the evidence which underpins an approach that sees spirituality as   171
a resource for resilience. In order to provide effective assessment nursing/midwifery   172
staff must understand the role beliefs can play in the human response to key life events   173
that may involve suffering or indeed joy. Working 'with the grain' of patients' spiritu-   174
ality has the potential to enable a deeper connection between clinician and patient   175
while allowing additional support, such as chaplaincy, to provide assistance.   176

While spiritual needs and their assessment can be complex, the initial explora-   177
tion with patients requires simplicity. For that reason, the EPICC Project adopted   178
the use of two questions (advocated by Ross and McSherry [12]) known as the   179
2QSAM. The questions enquire about what is most important to the patient and   180
invite the patient to inform the practitioner about what might be of help. It is person--   181
centred, colloquial and an open approach.   182

- *In the two case scenarios that follow, you will see how the 2QSAM has been*   183
  adapted and used in practice.   184

It is contrasted with other conversations in the clinical setting which may be   185
searching for specific answers in order to achieve a medical solution to a specific   186
problem. This open approach to spiritual assessment allows the patient to set the   187
agenda and identify the resources which may enable a better quality of life. For   188
example, a Muslim patient may be distressed that a clinical procedure may include   189
elements of care which run contrary to their beliefs, such as the offer of care by   190
someone who is not of the same gender as the patient. Identifying these beliefs and   191
the concerns they generate could allow care to be delivered in ways which are more   192
person-centred and reduce stress.   193

In summary, the assessment of spiritual need should be conducted in lan-   194
guage which is most comfortable for the patient. Technical terms or closed   195
questions are likely to reduce the candour with which personal beliefs are   196
shared. The humanity of the clinician and the open nature of questions can   197
begin a discussion which allows the patient to share issues of personal convic-   198
tion which may be both deeply personal and of assistance in helping them cope   199
with an episode of illness. Therefore, the attitudes, values and behaviours of the   200

201   professional undertaking the spiritual assessment are of paramount importance,
202   and these should always be sensitive to the cultural, ethnic and religious back-
203   ground of the person.

204   ## 7.4   The Need for Culturally Sensitive Care an Example
205   from Thailand

206   A great deal of the work undertaken and published around spirituality and spiritual
207   assessment has focused specifically on adult contexts and settings. Very little evi-
208   dence and practical resources are produced with children and young people in mind.
209   Additionally, much of the research published on spirituality and spiritual care origi-
210   nates from Western cultures.
211   In the following section, we introduce the concept of spiritual assessment with
212   adolescents providing an example from work undertaken with adolescents in
213   Thailand. The principle that spirituality is a universal concept and understood by all,
214   is being challenged within healthcare, especially from countries whose culture may
215   not have a word or language to define this dimension of the person. This is of impor-
216   tance when undertaking a spiritual assessment with individuals from different coun-
217   tries and cultures outside of the Western hemisphere.
218   Providing spiritual care or promoting spiritual well-being in the Thai context is
219   challenging due to several factors. The concept and term 'spirituality' that are used
220   may in the West may not be something Thai people in general and adolescents in
221   particular are familiar with. This is because the word spirituality and its translations
222   from English into Thai, are grounded in a different culture and religion. Western
223   understandings of spirituality are likely to be influenced by Christianity [13],
224   whereas the concept of spirituality to Thai people is influenced by Buddhism in
225   particular [14].
226   Bearing these cultural differences in mind when conducting research promoting
227   spiritual well-being for Thai adolescents, a simple question related to the concept of
228   spirituality was used to assess spiritual well-being. In the study the main questions
229   we asked were: (1) 'What is your purpose in life and How important is it to you',
230   and (2) 'What is the most important thing or most important person in your life?'
231   and (3) 'What do you want to do for them?'
232   This research recruited 21 adolescents aged 14–15 years (Buddhism and
233   Muslim). Each adolescent was asked either the first or second question above [15].
234   Most participants explained that their purpose in life was associated with their
235   desire for a positive future career. Some of the responses provided were related to
236   aims, quests and what to do in the future. They needed to make these happen, so
237   they would be able to live a good life. Many participants aimed to have good, secure
238   and honest occupations, so that they could support their parents and their benefac-
239   tors. Some of them knew that having a good occupation would make their parents
240   proud and happy and that would reflect their gratitude towards their parents. Three

participants wanted to be nurses because they perceived that nursing was a good and   241
secure occupation, and they could use their profession in caring for their parents and   242
people around them. As Pim, a junior high school girl who comes from a poor   243
socio-economic background explained. An example of the conversation is provided   244
in Box 7.3:   245

It was interesting to note that many of the participants identified themselves,   246
their parents, family members, friends and society in general as being the most   247
important persons in their life. In addition, with this increased awareness of the   248
value of themselves and significant others, their purpose in life seemed to be focused   249
upon doing good things for those very same people. Several responses received   250
from some of the adolescents are provided in Box 7.4:   251

Box 7.3 Conversation Between Dr. Balthip and Pim

Karnsunaphat: What is your purpose in life? (What would you like to be when you grow up?)

    Pim: *Having a goal to become a nurse is very meaningful to me. I can care for or treat myself, my parents, persons close to me.*

Karnsunaphat: You want to be a nurse because you want to care for your parents.

    Pim: *Yes, my parents look after me since I was young. I want to care for them... My parents have given me so much love, care and concern ever since I was young, I know I cannot find love like this anywhere else; it fills me with respect for them. I want to take care of them, and to try to make my life as successful as I can to make them feel proud of me. Every morning, I help my mother sell vegetables at the market. I want to help her as much as I can... My parents cared for me since I was born. They both work very hard to support our family. I want to pay them back by taking care of both of them.*

Box 7.4: Responses from Adolescents About What Was Important to Them

People who love themselves will have commitment to do good things in life not from a sense of duty but because they really want to. They pay attention to the things that will bring positivity to their life.

    My family economic status is not really good. My father has had a stroke. My older sister and mother have to take care of my father. I always want to present my gratitude to them by paying attention to my study. When I get a good score, my parents feels proud of me, this makes me feel happy.

    I feel proud of being Thai... We have our own land. We have the best king. So, I have to protect my country... As a Thai adolescent I have duties to do good things for my society. I have to have knowledge to develop my nation.

They also provided an example of how having a positive purpose in life was important to them. Many adolescents described the significance of having purpose in life and that having purpose in life was like having a direction. It was like a compass directing the way to move on. When they had a positive purpose in life, they knew what to do and what not to do. This purpose provided an opportunity to plan their future and instil a quest to achieve it. They aimed to have 'a good life or better life'. As a male adolescent explained:

> I am the eldest son. I need to inherit my father's business, so he won't have to work so hard. He has worked so hard. I think I need to study in a technical college so I can get the job I want without having to use the trial and error technique. [16]

So, these two simple, yet thought-provoking questions could potentially be highly valuable to all stakeholders working with adolescents. The questions are intended to bring into sharp focus for the adolescents those things which are of the utmost importance in their life and to stimulate them into thinking deeply about how they can discover and advance their own positive life path.

7.4.1 Explanation Applying Knowledge, Skills and Attitudes Evident in the Scenario

Spirituality is a broad concept comprising several attributes and characteristics including meaning and purpose in life, fulfilment, transcendence, connectedness, relationships also embracing religious concepts [17, 18]. In the adolescent context, one of the main attributes used and which is related to their growth and development trajectory [19] is purpose in life and connectedness. Therefore, the two main questions, mentioned above, focus primarily upon relationship, meaning and purpose in life. Box 7.5 applies the scenario and research to the knowledge, skills and attitudes required when assessing the spiritual needs of adolescents within a Thai context. However, the lessons learned from this exercise are transferrable into other contexts and situations.

The evidence suggests that spirituality plays a key significant role in the cultivation of good health, healing, and well-being [20]. A systematic review exploring the impact of adolescents' religiosity/spirituality and mental health found that most studies (90%) showed that adolescents who reported higher levels of religiosity/spirituality were more likely to report having better mental health [21]. The findings suggested that the majority of participants agreed that spirituality significantly affected their sense of wellness. They believed that spirituality is an important dimension of wellness that will lead to an increased level of self-esteem and helps provide a set of rules that can assist them to live a better or healthier life [22].

Box 7.5: Application to Knowledge, Skills and Attitudes

Knowledge	Skills	Attitudes	
Spirituality is the essence of life. During the course of the study, I deliberately avoided using the term spirituality as this term is not widely used in Thailand (as mentioned above). However, as spirituality is the essence of life, I wished to understand what was the essence of the respective participant's life by asking questions based upon guidance received from the work of McSherry et al. [11]. The questions being: 'What is the most important thing or most important person in your life?' and 'What do you want to do for them?'	Providing spiritual care does not need any kind of advanced technology. However, being able to provide spiritual care may not always be intuitive or innate This means as nursing and midwifery students, we may need to practice being compassionate. To gain an understanding of the attributes associated with the term spirituality, it is better to structure questions (as outlined above) around assessing their purpose in life. The two questions used in this scenario can be used with adolescents in both the clinical and non-clinical settings	The main attitudes which would ideally be found in nursing students for providing spiritual care to patients are: (1) recognise the significance of spirituality, (2) know that everyone has spirituality not only the end-of-life patients or patients in a critical condition, and (3) spirituality is not difficult to assess and support. It is about taking time to show compassion and empathy to the patient by touch, eye contact, smiling and listening with an empathetic and kind manner	t3.1 t3.2 t3.3 t3.4 t3.5 t3.6 t3.7 t3.8 t3.9 t3.10 t3.11 t3.12 t3.13 t3.14 t3.15 t3.16 t3.17 t3.18 t3.19 t3.20 t3.21 t3.22 t3.23 t3.24

Reflective Exercise 2

What do you think about providing or promoting the spiritual development of adolescents?

7.5   Importance of Self-Awareness When Planning Spiritual Care

The following section presents a scenario (Box 7.6) from the research undertaken   288
by Dr. Yanping Niu exploring the meaning and experiences of spirituality and spir-   289
itual care among people from Chinese backgrounds living in England [23]. The   290
reason for introducing you to this research is that it demonstrates the importance of   291
nurses, midwives and healthcare professionals being sensitive to the needs of peo-   292
ple from diverse cultures and communities. The scenario also highlights some key   293
issues about self-awareness and how this is important in maintaining personal and   294
professional boundaries. Having a high level of self-awareness is vitally important   295
when undertaking a spiritual assessment and when planning to deliver spiri-   296
tual care.   297
                                                                        298
                                                                        299

Box 7.6: Importance of Self-Awareness in Maintaining Personal and Professional Boundaries

I first met Lian at a Chinese Centre in the UK where I volunteered teaching English. Lian is from Fujian province in China. She visits the Centre regularly and participates in different social activities such as learning English, playing table tennis, going out with friends, and learning about Chinese opera. But her attendance at the English class was intermittent. One day, I had the opportunity to speak with her about her understanding of spiritual distress since she was a participant in my PhD research [23]. Before the conversation started, Lian provided me with some demographic information stating that she was an 'Atheist' and that she also followed 'Mixed Philosophies' [notice Lian seemed to follow several faiths or beliefs].

Yanping: Would you mind telling about your faith?

Lian: *Um... I do not have any faith. I am atheist.*

Yanping: What is important to you?

Lian: *I think when a person does things, he should follow his heart, and try his best to help others instead of hurting. He should assume his basic responsibility. Considering my situation, my husband does not take care of our children. But I still listen to his words so that my children could grow up in parental love. Family members living together is predetermined by heaven and their fate. My children came to us because of this. Since I gave birth to them and I would try my best to bring them up no matter what happens. Life is hard in UK because we cannot speak English and we do not have many friends.*

Yanping: Could you tell me more about it?

Lian: *My husband lost his business in China and came here 15 years ago. He did not want his acquaintances to know he has nothing. After arriving he found things were not as what he had thought, and he could not find a job. This is because he cannot speak English and had no friends to help. He then started to gamble since he had no family around and he can communicate with people in gambling place. To prevent him from becoming a compulsive gambler, I came to accompany him. Every weekend when he does not work, he gambles. I used to call him back and accompany him during weekend. Now I leave him alone. I cannot stop him from gambling no matter how hard I tried.*

Yanping: This is sad.

Lian: *In the past 2 years, I have sought help from a psychiatrist. I was sued for mistreating old people in care home. A group of colleagues provided false accusation against me. I could not defend myself because I could not speak English. I had been very kind in helping others but had lost motivation in doing so because of this. I am frightened and unable to control my thought since then. I do not understand why this happens to me. My suffering is predetermined. It is my fate. An old Chinese saying says 'Heaven is watching what a person is doing' so I think the justice will eventually come to me. The diffi-culties may make me stronger.*

[When she describes her issues, her eyes are full of tears. I hold her hands to comfort her.]

Yanping: Do you think a faith, such as Buddhism, can somehow help you?

Lian: *I am an atheist and I believe that Gods, fairies and Buddha exist. Many Chinese people say that fairy and Buddha are within me, but I am still suffering so badly.*

[notice Lian claims she is an atheist but believes that Gods, fairies and Buddha exist].

Yanping: What are your expectations of spiritual care?

Lian: *My current focus is to recover from the illness and difficult situation, I do not care about spiritual care.*

[As a nurse or healthcare professional how might you respond to this situation and identify needs?]

The interview was scheduled for about 1 h, but the conversation lasted for about 2 h. I realised that Lian has spiritual needs and allowed her to set the pace so that we could explore her spiritual concerns.

7.5.1 Explanation Applying Knowledge, Skills and Attitudes Evident in the Scenario

The cultural care theory, Culture Care and Universality [24], highlights the importance of an individual's values, beliefs and contextual factors such as relationships, finance and political considerations. Keeping these considerations in mind guided Dr. Niu's assessment and ensured this was conducted in a culturally sensitive manner.

The spiritual assessment in the scenario generally followed an integration of Faith and belief Importance, Community and Address in care tool [25] and Two Question Spiritual/holistic Assessment Model (2QSAM): The power of two simple questions [12]. The first question 'What is your faith or belief?' was modified by Dr. Niu to 'Would you mind telling about your faith?' This question did not elicit valuable information regarding spiritual care. This may be because many people who have an affiliation to a particular faith generally do not discuss it openly in Chinese culture. Dr. Niu then used the question 'What is important to you?' from the 2QSAM to make further evaluation. Lian articulated the stress she had experienced in her family. She also indicated that her children could be a source of support, and Buddhist philosophy explains her fate and suffering. Realising the power of this question, Dr. Niu used it again by asking 'Could you tell me more about it?' Lian elaborated informing her about the recent stress she had encountered during a legal case. Because she kept referring to this issue, it was probably more relevant to her than her family problems. During the conversation, Lian showed the sign of

321 distress, such as worry, crying, 'why this happen to me'. This signifies she had some
322 deep emotional and spiritual needs [26].
323   The second question Dr. Niu asked from FICA was regarding the importance of
324 faith, which was slightly reworded to 'What role do these beliefs play?' to 'Do you
325 think a faith, such as Buddhism, can somehow help you?' Dr. Niu asked this ques-
326 tion because she had explained that her experiences in family are destined and pre-
327 determined by heaven and her fate. This is very similar to Buddhism teachings. Lian
328 did not indicate she needed support with her faith but emphasised again the current
329 issue she faced with her job. Since she has no need for support with a particular
330 faith, Dr. Niu refrained from asking the third question in FICA 'Are you part of a
331 spiritual and religious community?'
332   After realising that what bothered or concerned her most was issues associated
333 with her employment, Dr. Niu let Lian dictate the pace of the interview (Giske and
334 Cone 2015) before introducing the fourth question in FICA and 2QSAM 'How can
335 I help?' Lian then asked Dr. Niu to help with her language barriers that she was
336 experiencing. By being open to her request, Dr. Niu was willing to offer some sup-
337 port during this time of emotional turmoil, signposting her to relevant avenues of
338 support.
339   Through the above assessment, Dr. Niu identified Lian's primary spiritual need
340 was associated with securing employment to overcome the trouble she is currently
341 facing. Her children were a strong support throughout this crisis. During the assess-
342 ing process, Dr. Niu became aware of the importance of engaging other professions
343 in providing spiritual care. For example, if Lian indicated she needed support within
344 the Buddhist tradition, then it might have been appropriate to introduce her to a
345 priest from the local Buddhist community. Also, Dr. Niu could advise Lian to attend
346 some support group to help with translations. All these referrals would need to be
347 done with Lian's consent. Dr. Niu describes another important aspect of spiritual
348 assessment that is dealing with emotions by holding her hands, showing empathy by
349 using words such as 'This is sad'. Being open to her requests and listening atten-
350 tively to her response to the question 'How can I help?' demonstrated a willingness
351 to be present with her during this very emotionally turbulent and difficult time [3].
352   Before proceeding with the remainder of the chapter it would be useful to spend
353 a few moments reflecting on some of the key points raised in Dr. Niu's scenario and
354 how these might apply to your own professional practice.

Reflective Exercise 3
When Dr Niu saw Lian's eyes full of tears, she did not do anything but kept asking questions. Do you think this was appropriate?

When Dr Niu recognised Lian had a faith, belief in Chinese philosophy when she stated, 'fairy and Buddha are within me", do you think it was appropriate for Dr Niu to introduce her to a Buddhist faith community?

Was Dr Niu correct in suggesting this?

Box 7.7: Application to Knowledge, Skills and Attitudes

Knowledge	Skill	Attitudes	
Many different spiritual assessment tools are available. In this scenario, I have only applied knowledge from FICA [25] and 2QSAM [12] I also demonstrate knowledge about the different social care and faith groups that are present in this particular Chinese community, to which I can refer Lian [27] I understand that the meaning of spiritual care might be different in Chinese culture. Chinese values, belief, contextual factor such as relationships, finance and political considerations shape Lian's spiritual needs I understand the need to gain Lian's consent for referral (EPPIC 2019) and support to other agencies or groups [3]	I demonstrate the ability to use different spiritual assessment tools and am aware how these may be helpful in specific situations I recognise sign of spiritual distress, such as worry, crying, complaining 'Why has this happened to me' (Giske and Cone 2015), and follow up on these signs of distress. This is done by using open-questions 'Tell me more about it', holding Lian's hand, speaking to her using kind, compassionate words, validating her feeling for example 'This is sad', allowing the pace of the assessment to be determined by Lian's needs (Giske and Cone 2015) I gain consent to refer Lian for social support. Being sensitive to Lian's response relating to Chinese culture, such as why Lian's faith is contradictory [23]? Why the first question did not elicit relevant information? Why she says her suffering is her fate? Why Lian says she does not need spiritual care?	Being open to Lian's request by asking open-ended questions such as 'how can I help?' and willing to offer emotional and psychological support during this very stressful time	t4.1 t4.2 t4.3 t4.4 t4.5 t4.6 t4.7 t4.8 t4.9 t4.10 t4.11 t4.12 t4.13 t4.14 t4.15 t4.16 t4.17 t4.18 t4.19 t4.20 t4.21 t4.22 t4.23 t4.24 t4.25 t4.26 t4.27 t4.28 t4.29 t4.30 t4.31 t4.32 t4.33 t4.34 t4.35

7.6   Why Spiritual Assessment Matters: Thoughts from a Newly Qualified Nurse

This final section has been written by Sarah McKay who was a final year student when she took part in the EPICC Project studying Adult Nursing at Liverpool University in England, United Kingdom.

7.6.1   Why It Matters?

Spirituality is unique to each human being. It is at the core of our identity, shaping
how we make sense of and draw meaning from our lives. Spirituality is central to our
relationships and guides us in how we face challenges. Illness is but one of these
challenges and therefore it is important as nurses and healthcare professionals to be
able to identify patients spirituality and highlight their needs. Spiritual assessment is
all about listening to a patient and their relatives, devoting time to draw on what will
bring them hope and courage during times of suffering and uncertainty [28].
Therefore, it is not defined by a set of check boxes or structured plan, it is a conversation in which the nurse or midwife is looking to truly find the person in the patient [29].

7.6.2   Developing Patient Awareness

Developing patient awareness of spirituality through spiritual assessment has lots to
add to a patient journey, whether this be a single admission into hospital or multiple.
Patients recognise this when a healthcare professional is seeking to care for their
'whole' person [30]. As human beings, to feel valued and have your needs acknowledged is heart-warming and reassuring to know that there are others looking out for
you and what you personally care about. Spiritual assessment also looks to motivate
patients by increasing their awareness of what they can lean on in tough times and
allow them to draw strength from that. Inspiring courage is a crucial part of the
recovery process [28].

7.6.3   Demonstrating Spiritual Care

One way I feel this is demonstrated in the NHS is through the role of the specialist
nurse. In a local NHS cancer hospital, specialist nurses provide a service to those
living with the cancer to which they are a specialist in. Patients can build rapport
with their specialist nurse, through appointments and contact if ever admitted in
hospital. This role serves patients spirituality as specialist nurse can really get to
know their patients, have time through several appointments to assess their spiritual
as well as their medical needs and is a point of contact for them to turn to during
difficulties. The holistic nature of the role gives patients an opportunity to discuss
current and potential treatment as well as plans for the future. The nurse is then able
to act as an advocate for the patient along with any relatives.

Spirituality as well as being an integral part of nursing care is also an integral part
of being a nurse and midwife. As a newly qualified nurse, it is easy to be critical of
the care we provide, as learning is constant and there is so much to think of and
remember. It is overwhelming, as you are now fully responsible for the care of your

patients rather than being supported by a mentor. It is so different from being a student, as although you are surrounded by supportive staff, you question yourself on things that you did not question as a student.

There is a lot of time pressures to adhere to, and in the first few months, it has been important to learn how to effectively deal with them. It is important to care for our own spirituality as people as well as being nurses, by identifying methods to combat stress and pressure, some examples being hobbies, sports, family and faith. And so, highlighting what brings meaning and purpose in our own lives can enhance our vocation as nurses as by caring for ourselves we are then more equipped to be able to holistically care for patients [31].

As a newly qualified nurse, in the business and chaos of a 12-h shift, at times it feels like awareness of spirituality and assessment have been lost. However, on reflection, spirituality is ingrained in care despite a lack of awareness of it. Spirituality is an attitude which we all possess when we value others and look to support them.

Building on this attitude with further awareness of spirituality is important because:

- Learning from experiences.
- Spiritual assessment, learning to properly listen to people.
- Assessment is more than just listening to a patient's or relative's word; it is also about their emotions and body language. This in turn serves patient and relatives spirituality and reinforces the importance of spirituality in the nurse.

7.7 Summary of the Main Points for Learning

This chapter has provided an overview of some of the key approaches to spiritual assessment that can be used within nursing and midwifery practice. The scenarios demonstrate the importance of having a high degree of self-awareness and how this is essential in preserving the personal and professional boundaries that exist. Implicitly throughout the chapter the benefits of supporting the spiritual needs of those receiving care are outlined. Nurses and midwives being human and providing care for other humans as patients, mothers, carers, brings a special quality to care. Although this may present nursing and midwifery with some challenges, personally and professionally, it brings many positives when working with and looking after people, as both a nurse and human being can empathise.

Competence and confidence in the area of spiritual assessment can be acquired at many levels and through many activities. However, as nurses or midwifes, we must constantly strive for excellence in caring for people's spirituality, and this can only be achieved through competent assessment having sound underpinning knowledge in conjunction with the correct attitudes, behaviours and skills. Yet, this must be balanced with an understanding that any expectations around the comprehensiveness of this are realistic and attainable. It is not so much about being an expert but about demonstrating sensitivity rather than ignorance. It is about being informed, knowing one's own limitations and seeking, actively engaging the support of other professionals when necessary.

Spiritual assessment takes many forms; irrespective of the approach used, this must always be undertaken in a relationship that is based on mutual trust, understanding, with clear lines of consent, responding to the needs of the person in a holistic, compassionate and ethical manner.

References

1. EPICC Spiritual Care Education Standard (2019). Available from http://blogs.staffs.ac.uk/epicc/resources-and-tools/epicc-spiritual-care-education-standard. [Accessed 19-03-2021]
2. Stoll R. Guidelines for spiritual assessment. Am J Nurs. 1979;1:1572–7.
3. McSherry W. Spiritual assessment: definition, categorisation and features. In: McSherry W, Ross L, editors. Spiritual assessment in healthcare practice. Keswick: M&K Update; 2010.
4. Bernard M, Strasser F, Gamondi C, Braunschweig G, Forster M, Kaspers-Elekes K, Veri SW, Borasio GD, Pralong G, Pralong J, Marthy S. Relationship between spirituality, meaning in life, psychological distress, wish for hastened death, and their influence on quality of life in palliative care patients. J Pain Symptom Manage. 2017;54(4):514–22.
5. Park K, Henderson J. "The first hospital among Christians": the ospedale di Santa Maria Nuova in early sixteenth-century Florence. Med Hist. 1991;35(2):164–88.
6. Monod S, Brennan M, Rochat E, Martin E, Rochat S, Büla CJ. Instruments measuring spirituality in clinical research: a systematic review. J Gen Intern Med. 2011 Nov;26(11):1345-57. https://doi.org/10.1007/s11606-011-1769-7. Epub 2011 Jul 2. PMID: 21725695; PMCID: PMC3208480.
7. Peterman AH, Reeve CL, Winford EC, Cotton S, Salsman JM, McQuellon R, Tsevat J, Campbell C. Measuring meaning and peace with the FACIT–spiritual well-being scale: distinction without a difference? Psychol Assess. 2014;26(1):127.
8. Vlasblom JP, Van Der Steen JT, Walton MN, Jochemsen H. Effects of nurses' screening of spiritual needs of hospitalized patients on consultation and perceived nurses' support and patients' spiritual well-being. Holist Nurs Pract. 2015;29(6):346–56.
9. Harvey K, Brown B, Crawford P, Candlin S. "Elicitation hooks": a discourse analysis of chaplain-patient interaction in pastoral and spiritual care. J Pastoral Care Counsel. 2008;62(1–2):43–61.
10. McSherry W, Ross L. Dilemmas of spiritual assessment: considerations for nursing practice. J Adv Nurs. 2002;38(5):479–88.
11. McSherry W, Ross L, Balthip K., Ross N., & Young S. Spiritual assessment in healthcare—an overview of comprehensive, sensitive approaches to spiritual assessment for use within the interdisciplinary healthcare team. In: Timmins F, Caldeira S, editors. Spirituality in healthcare: quality and performance. Berlin: Springer Nature; 2019.
12. Ross L, McSherry W. The power of two simple questions. Nurs Stand. 2018;33(9):78–80.
13. Sheldrake P. A brief history of spirituality. Victoria: Blackwell Publishing. 2007.
14. Tongprateep T. Spiritual care: nursing process. The Thai Journal of Nursing Council. 2002;17(1):1–12.
15. Balthip K, Petchruschatachart U, Piriyakoontorn S, Liamputtong P. Purpose in life among Thai junior high school adolescents. Songklanagarind J Nurs. 2017a;37(Supplement):89–97.
16. Balthip Q, Petchruschatachart P. Spiritual care for patients living with chronic health condition in the community. Songkhla: P.C. prospect. (Thai); 2016.

17. Balthip K, McSherry W, Petchruschatachart P, Piriyakoontorn S, Liamputtong P. Enhancing life purpose amongst Thai adolescents. J Moral Educ. 2017b;46(3):295–307. https://doi.org/10.1080/03057240.2017.1347089.

18. Puchalski CM, Vitillo R, Hull SK, Reller N. Improving the spiritual dimension of whole person care: reaching national and international consensus. J Palliat Med. 2014;17(6):642–56. https://doi.org/10.1089/jpm.2014.9427. Epub 2014 May 19. PMID: 24842136; PMCID: PMC4038982.

19. Sawyer SM, Afifi RA, Bearinger LH, Blakemore SJ, Dick B, Ezeh AC, Patton GC. Adolescence: a foundation for future health. Lancet. 2012;379(9826):1630–40.

20. Koenig H, King D, Carson VB. Handbook of Religion and Health (2nd Ed) Oxford University Press, Oxford. 2002.

21. Wong YJ, Rew L, Slaikeu KD. A systematic review of recent research on adolescent religiosity/spirituality and mental health. Issues Mental Health Nursing, 2006;27(2):161–83.

22. Spurr S, Berry L, Walker K. The meanings older adolescents attach to spirituality Journal for Specialists in Pediatric Nursing. 2013;18:221–23.

23. Niu Y. Meaning and experiences of spirituality and spiritual care among people from Chinese backgrounds living in England: a grounded theory investigation. PhD Thesis. Staffordshire University; 2019.

24. Mcfarland MR. Madeline Leininger: cultural care theory of diversity and universality. In ALLIGOOD, M. R. &MARRINER-TOMEY, A. (eds.) Nursing Theorists and Their Work. 8th ed. London: Mosby. 2014.

25. Puchalski C, Romer AL. Taking a spiritual history allows clinicians to understand patients more fully. J Palliat Med. 2000;3(1):129–37.

26. Giske T. Cone PH. Discerning the healing path – how nurses assist patient spirituality in diverse health care settings. Journal of Clinical Nursing. 2015;24:(19-20). p. 2926–35.

27. Puchalski C. The spiritual history: an essential element of patient-centred care. In: McSherry W, Ross L, editors. Spiritual assessment in healthcare practice. Keswick: M&K Update; 2010.

28. Baldacchino D. Spiritual care education of healthcare professionals. Religions. 2015;6(2):594–613.

29. Nursing and Midwifery Council. The Code: professional standards of practice and behaviour for nurses and midwives. 2018. https://www.nmc.org.uk/globalassets/sitedocuments/nmc-publications/nmc-code.pdf Accessed 30 Mar 2020.

30. Cooper K, Chang E. Undergraduate nursing student's perspectives of spiritual care education in an Australian context. Nurse Educ Today. 2016;44:74–8.

31. Paparella G. Understanding staff wellbeing, its impact on patient experience and health-care quality. 2015. http://www.picker.org/wp-content/uploads/2015/06/2015-06-10-StaffWellbeingBriefing.Pdf. Accessed 1 Dec 2019.

Suggested Reading

Read the Chapter McSherry W, Ross L, Balthip K, Ross N, Young S. Spiritual assessment in healthcare- an overview of comprehensive, sensitive approaches to spiritual assessment for use within the interdisciplinary healthcare team. In: Timmins F, Caldeira S, editors. Spirituality in healthcare: perspectives for innovative practice. Cham: Springer Nature; 2019.

Read section 'Communication about spiritual issues' and 'Stages in assessing spiritual issues' in Puchalski, C. The spiritual history: an essential element of patient-centred care. In: McSherry W, Ross L, editors. Spiritual assessment in healthcare practice. Keswick: M&K Update Ltd.; 2010.

Read section 'Turning on spirituality' in recognising the signs for spiritual distress and 'Following the patient's pace' in Giske T, Cone PH. Discerning the healing path—how nurses assist patient spirituality in diverse health care settings. J Clin Nurs. 2015;24(19–20):2926–35.

Chapter 8
Competence 4: Spiritual Care, Intervention and Evaluation

Tove Giske, Aliza Damsma-Bakker, Sílvia Caldeira, Gracia M. González-Romero, Wilson C. de Abreu, and Fiona Timmins

Learning Objectives

This chapter will enable you to:

1. Reflect on how to provide spiritual care interventions demonstrating compassion, presence, empathy, openness, professional humility and trustworthiness.
2. Know how to plan spiritual interventions by identifying appropriate resources; along with responding to, evaluating and documenting how spiritual needs have been met.
3. Reflect on personal spiritual care competencies and personal limitations, and how to manage these in a professional way, including referring to others as appropriate.

T. Giske (✉)
Faculty of Health Studies, VID Specialized University, Bergen, Norway
e-mail: tove.giske@vid.no

A. Damsma-Bakker
Faculty of Health Care, Viaa University of Applied Science, Zwolle, The Netherlands
e-mail: a.damsma@viaa.nl

S. Caldeira
Institute of Health Sciences, Centre for Interdisciplinary Research in Health,
Universidade Católica Portuguesa, Lisbon, Portugal
e-mail: scaldeira@ucp.pt

G. M. González-Romero
Servicio Madrileño de Salud (SERMAS), Comunidad de Madrid, Madrid, Spain

W. C. de Abreu
Porto School of Nursing, Center for Health Technology and Services Research,
University of Porto, Porto, Portugal
e-mail: wjabreu@esenf.pt

F. Timmins
School of Nursing and Midwifery, Trinity College, Dublin, Irland
e-mail: timminsf@tcd.ie

© Springer Nature Switzerland AG 2021
W. McSherry et al. (eds.), *Enhancing Nurses' and Midwives' Competence in Providing Spiritual Care*, https://doi.org/10.1007/978-3-030-65888-5_8

8.1   Introduction

This chapter builds upon your learning from previous chapters, and in particular Chap. 7, where fundamental principles and practices regarding spiritual assessment and the planning of spiritual care were outlined. This chapter aims to guide on how spiritual care interventions may be chosen and developed once spiritual assessment has taken place. These spiritual care interventions are provided in the context of EPICC spiritual care competency 4 (Table 8.1). To support your understanding of these interventions, and how these might work in clinical practice, we provide four case studies that are explained and discussed within the chapter.

We will focus on what the provision of spiritual care interventions to patients in practice realistically means in terms of demands from nurses and midwives, both professionally and personally. This chapter will explore different ways spiritual care can be (a) addressed and evaluated, and (b) documented in nursing and midwifery. By using the four case studies, this chapter provides clear and practical information on spiritual care interventions including necessary documentation, and how to evaluate these interventions. The chapter is organised according to the three key learning objectives stated earlier.

Spirituality is widely recognised as an important consideration in modern healthcare, and there is convincing evidence that many patients and their families have spiritual needs and resources that, if addressed within healthcare, contribute to the provision of optimal care [1]. Certainly, the EPICC project (2016–2019), upon which this book is based, gained consensus internationally from both clinicians and patients, that spirituality is a fundamental aspect of healthcare. Understanding what constitutes both spirituality and spiritual care is outlined in Chap. 2, and the present chapter is concerned with actions arising from expressed spiritual needs and resources that inform spiritual care delivery within the context of a caring compassionate relationship (Table 8.1). A more detailed understanding of spiritual intervention will now be provided.

Table 8.1 Competence 4: Spiritual Care: Intervention and Evaluation   t1.1

Responds to spiritual needs and resources within a caring, compassionate relationship			t1.2
Knowledge (cognitive)	Skills (functional)	Attitudes (behavioural)	t1.3
– Understands the concept of compassion and presence and its importance in spiritual care – Knows how to respond appropriately to identified spiritual needs and resources – Knows how to evaluate whether spiritual needs have been met	– Recognises personal limitations in spiritual care giving and refers to others as appropriate – Evaluates and documents personal, professional and organisational aspects of spiritual care giving, and reassess appropriately	– Shows compassion and presence – Shows willingness to collaborate with and refer to others (professional/nonprofessional) – Is welcoming and accepting and shows empathy, openness, professional humility and trustworthiness in seeking additional spiritual support	t1.4 t1.5 t1.6 t1.7 t1.8 t1.9 t1.10 t1.11 t1.12 t1.13 t1.14 t1.15 t1.16 t1.17

8.1.1   What Is a Spiritual Intervention?

Nurses and midwives are expected to identify spiritual needs and resources, to plan
effective interventions, to evaluate the health outcomes and to document and record
that process. The primary requirement within this competence framework is to
respond to a patient's spiritual needs and resources within a caring and compassionate relationship. Thus, relationship building with patients and their families is a key
competence for all nurses and midwives in providing spiritual interventions.
Beyond this, the nurse/midwife must understand the concepts of compassion and
presence because having these skills facilitates the provision of spiritual care.
Having compassion and being present are spiritual interventions [2]. The nurse/
midwife must also know how to respond appropriately to a person's identified spiritual needs and resources and understand how to evaluate whether or not spiritual
needs have been met and the patient's/client's resources utilised. Resources to support the nurse and midwife with these tasks will be discussed and outlined in this
chapter; however, it is essential to learn, understand and be aware of personal
boundaries.

   This approach requires that the nurses/midwives understand the concepts of
compassion and presence (Table 8.1) and how these fit within a framework of spiritual care. Spiritual care is understood as care that responds in a human way to others, especially when facing life-altering events (such as birth, trauma and ill health)
or sadness [3]. As such, the core aspect of spiritual care is emphasising a human
dimension of care and the importance of relationships, based on compassion and
empathy, offered through presence and inspiring trust [4]. For some patients, spiritual care, and providing interventions related to this, will occur through the relationship. This is one that is supportive and compassionate, provides a listening ear and
allows the person to express their fears, needs and desires. Indeed, 'spiritual care
begins with encouraging human contact in a compassionate relationship and moves
in whatever direction need requires' (NHS Scotland [3]. For others, spiritual care
requires a support of their personal faith or beliefs, perhaps requiring referral to
healthcare chaplain or spiritual advisor to receive support with faith rituals or prayer.

   Within the process of this competence, it is clear that the nurse/midwife must
recognise their personal limitations in providing spiritual care (Table 8.1) and refer
to specialists when required. While the nurse/midwife is a key resource for supporting spiritual care and should be trained and aware in relation to interventions that
support spiritual care, patients' well-being and dignity, in many healthcare settings
internationally there are specialist spiritual advisors, such as healthcare chaplains,
who can support patients and their family directly. Being aware of the ethical boundaries of spiritual care is critical. Sometimes you may be able to provide direct care,
if for example a patient requests to share their hopes and fears with you in conversation. However, if for example their request concerns complex family relations and
difficulty with forgiveness, you might consider, with the patient's permission, referring to another healthcare professional who is more competent to help patients with
such spiritual needs. Spiritual interventions are understood as intimate, individual

77   and important dimensions of care for many patients receiving healthcare, particu-
78   larly those facing critical or traumatic events [5]. The theory, rationale and evidence
79   for spiritual care interventions will now be discussed.

80   ## 8.2   Theory, Rationale and Evidence

81   ### 8.2.1   *Personal Competencies in Spiritual Care*

82   Spiritual care requires professional skills and attitudes that may exist intrinsically as
83   personal qualities, but importantly, they can be learned and honed as competencies
84   in providing spiritual care [6]. These attitudes include compassion, presence, to be
85   welcoming, open and accepting, and to show empathy, professional humility and
86   trustworthiness. From the EPICC Spiritual Care Education Standard [7], derived
87   from both evidence and a consensus approach, the required attitudes are articulated
88   as follows:

89   • Shows compassion and presence.
90   • Shows willingness to collaborate with and refer to others (professional/
91   non-professional).
92   • Is welcoming and accepting and shows empathy, openness, professional humil-
93   ity and trustworthiness in seeking additional spiritual support.

94   While exhibiting these competencies and attitudes does not necessarily guaran-
95   tee spiritual care, these are a prerequisite for spiritual care. Indeed, the definition of
96   spiritual care used in the EPICC Spiritual Care Education Standard ([7], p. 2) stan-
97   dard states 'spiritual care begins with encouraging human contact in compassionate
98   relationship'. Human connection and building relationships is considered an essen-
99   tial interpersonal competence and, quite outside of spiritual care, is understood as
100   the first step in providing a spiritual care intervention.
101   The nurse or midwife displaying *compassion* within the relationship is a crucial
102   spiritual intervention. Having *compassion* and providing *compassionate care* are
103   understood as essential components of modern nursing and midwifery, and compas-
104   sionate care is understood internationally as making time, being there, going the
105   extra mile, defending and advocacy, and personalization of care [8]. It should be
106   noted that compassion is not the same as *empathy*, as empathy is the ability to emo-
107   tionally put oneself in someone else's place, whereas compassion also requires
108   *action* following this emotional connection. Compassion could therefore be said to
109   be *empathy in action*.
110   *Presence* is the ability to simply to be with the other person in a quiet way that
111   provides the feeling of intense, uninterrupted attention, where the patient is the
112   focus of attention. Being present is also a competence and skill that can be acquired.
113   During time spent with patients and family, however short, you can give a sense of
114   importance to the other that displays this presence. When you display presence, you
115   aim to give your full attention; with good eye contact and calm facial expression,

not to appear distracted, or in a hurry to leave, and you demonstrate evidence that   116
you have heard what is said or acknowledge arising needs. Interestingly, a theory of   117
presence was developed by Baart [9] in the Netherlands, as a result of observations   118
of the work of priests and pastors who worked in the most challenging of situations.   119
Importantly, these were situations where there was often nothing left that could be   120
done to improve situations, or where practical interventions would not resolve the   121
problem or provide a solution to the complex problems people faced. Ultimately,   122
presence was exposed as a practice where a professional relates to the other person   123
with attention and dedication [9]. The person first tries to understand the true mean-   124
ing of the situation and the other person's needs; then reflects on how the other   125
person expresses their need for them, and only then progresses to planning and   126
providing care accordingly [9]. These principles are useful for nurses and midwives,   127
who are starting to learn or understand the skill of presence. Presence may be sum-   128
marised as paying attention, seeking to understand, reflecting on this understanding   129
and then taking action. In midwifery, this is well understood and embedded in the   130
philosophical phrase 'being with the woman' [10]. In the more acute and fast-paced   131
setting, the act of presence might require some development. This may mean a   132
reorientation away from the major focus being on healthcare priorities and tasks,   133
and more towards prioritising the patient and family and listening to their needs and   134
resources. While presence is understood as a key component of interpersonal skills   135
in many healthcare areas, presence in the context of spiritual care is particularly   136
focused on and respectful to spiritual dimensions of the personal or family needs.   137

8.2.2 Spiritual Intervention: Presence   138

Experts on the topic have highlighted *presence* as one of the three interventions (the   139
others include the use of words and actions) to support patients spiritually [2, 11].   140
Sometimes just one of these interventions may be effective; sometimes all three are   141
required, depending on the patient's individual situation.   142

Presence means to be authentically attentive and fully present when we are with   143
the patient or family. It means to be sensitive and to listen actively to what is   144
expressed verbally and non-verbally. It might mean to tolerate silence, show com-   145
passion, accept one's own and the other's vulnerability and engage in the situation   146
[2, 11]. Presence in the context of spiritual interventions may have a more expansive   147
meaning. For example, a patient may request a nurse or midwife to stay with them   148
while they pray or to help them find or assemble their religious items. Presence in   149
this context means being comfortable to be with the patient during such activity, and   150
not resisting it on the grounds of having a different faith or no faith. This support is   151
not the same as a nurse initiating faith rituals; rather it is supporting a person with a   152
ritual of comfort, in the same way that one might support other personal interests.   153
Thus, being present to a patient's faith ritual, if needed or requested, is a way of   154
using a patient's and family's resources in providing quality care and may be an   155
important intervention in some practice areas. Certainly, displaying great resistance   156
or ridiculing the patient or family would not be appropriate.   157

8.2.3 Spiritual Intervention: Words

Spiritual interventions include the use of words [2, 11]. *The use of words* can be of great help to patients and their families. That might mean engaging the patient in conversation, along with encouraging them to share and discuss important life events, their thoughts, emotions and experiences related to these. It is important within the context of spiritual care to find out what is important to patients and their families, to understand what they value and see as important in life. For some patients, speaking with healthcare professionals can be a source of support as they are often new relationships that sit outside of the family structure, and as such can provide opportunities to share concerns more openly. For some patients, the use of written words from sacred texts from their faith tradition can be of great help in times of need. Hymnbooks, devotional books or religious books such as the Bible, the Koran and others can bring hope and comfort in times of spiritual distress. Prayer can also be a powerful tool to ease spiritual pain. Sensitivity of the person's prayer tradition is important so the prayer can be carried out, silently, or aloud in a way that the patient finds supportive. Some of these uses of words can therefore be carried forward as actions.

8.2.4 Spiritual Intervention: Actions

Spiritual interventions include definitive *actions* [2, 11] based on individual patient needs and resources assessment (Chap. 7). Spiritual care often involves different actions so that care can be in accordance with the values and faith traditions of patients. All spiritual care should always be carried out with respect, sensitivity and permission from the patients. The UK Royal College of Nursing ([12], p. 9) provides the following advice to nurses and midwives before taking any action:

- Has the intervention been initiated by the patient/client?
- Has clear consent been given?
- Does it comply with your professional codes of practice?
- Does it comply with your employer's codes of practice?
- Is it safe and appropriate?
- Is it likely to cause offence?
- Do you feel comfortable?
- Do you have sufficient knowledge and skills?
- Is there adequate support and supervision for you and your patient/client?

Within this context, building on a brief spiritual screening such as those outlined in Chap. 7, you may find that there are some actions that you can implement to support patients and families in your care. This will likely be quite individualised, as this is the nature of spiritually; therefore, it is important to keep an open-mind and avoid assumptions. Such assumptions can be problematic as peoples' religious needs and requirements, even within a single faith tradition, vary tremendously. Ultimately, it is important to seek to understand each person and family within a framework of person-centred care. These individual needs can then form the basis of a spiritual care plan. Symbols and rituals, for example, are consistently important for people during challenging times, irrespective of whether or not the person is actively practising a faith. For example, lighting candles and singing could emerge as requirements in the provision of spiritual care. Specifically, there are rituals around death that vary according to cultural and religious traditions that many people may like to carry out, or perhaps not, again depending on individual needs. Other practical things related to nursing care may be use of symbolic clothing and the importance of covering certain parts of the body. These religious requirements are very important to patients and family when receiving healthcare. It is worth remembering that the solace and comfort found in symbols and rituals during difficult times, such as death, are not necessarily the prevail of the religious and for many have a cultural, historical tradition that transcends religious faith.

It is always best to *ask* and *assess* to find out in one or more questions where the patient is at. As Florence Nightingale said, 'how few there are who, by five or six pointed questions, can elicit the whole case and get accurately to know and be able to report *where* the patient is' ([13], p. 61). It is also helpful if your local healthcare practice provides some guidance on religious, non-religious and cultural practices that are relevant within the healthcare context such as the Intercultural Guide [14] provided by the health service in the Republic of Ireland. Of note, this reference guide is supported by an *Intercultural Health Strategy* which identified the need for:

> …culturally competent service provision … where service users from diverse backgrounds have specific cultural and religious needs around healthcare. Aspects of personal care and hygiene, spiritual beliefs and practices, and dietary needs are of particular relevance in this regard. Accommodation of such diverse needs in inpatient facilities is a key component of competence in responding to intercultural needs. ([15], p. 63)

Thus, we see overlap between cultural, religious and spiritual needs. Similarly, in Canada, the College of Nurses of Ontario published practice guidelines on culturally sensitive care [16] that included four elements of providing culturally sensitive care outlined as:

- Acquiring cultural knowledge.
- Facilitating client choice.
- Communication.
- Self-reflection.

Overall, determining a patient's and family's needs can be carried out in a straightforward manner as identified in Chap. 7, and central to this is good communication and asking the patient and family what their needs are. The potential variance of cultural, religious and personal plurality of needs both within individuals and within families are far too complex for a nurse or midwife to simply know. Acquiring cultural knowledge takes many approaches. While published guidelines and resources are useful, the most important resource is the patient and their family.

239 Therefore, determining the actions to support spiritual needs and utilise their
240 resources will require an individualised approach. It might require making sure that
241 the food choice is right. For some patients, it is imperative to have a vegetarian diet.
242 For others, it can be significant that they can eat special items. Solitude related to
243 prayer can be important for some, and for Muslims dependant on staying in bed, the
244 direction of the bed towards Mecca is imperative. Some religions have strict rules
245 for relationships between men and women that might influence nursing care and
246 medical investigations. Rituals related to washing the dead body is another signifi-
247 cant action with deep meaning for many people, and it can be essential that it is done
248 in the right way and of the right person. These religious requirements are very
249 important to patients and family when receiving healthcare and need respect, care-
250 ful assessment and action to ensure patient and family well-being.

251   A last action we will mention is the willingness and ability to refer to others as
252 needed. This action incorporates the skills that recognises personal limitations in
253 spiritual care-giving and leads to willingness to collaborate with and refer to others
254 (Table 8.1). This requires skills of self-reflection as have been identified above.
255 Indeed, the RCN also provides advice for nurses and midwives if they feel 'out of
256 their depth' ([12], p. 10). They suggest that it is about 'knowing your strengths,
257 limitations and when to seek help' ([12], p. 10). They suggest considering contact-
258 ing other people for support in these circumstances such as the following:

259 • Another colleague, someone you trust (mentor or preceptor).
260 • The healthcare chaplaincy team (who are there for staff and patients of all faiths
261   and none).
262 • Local contacts specific to your workplace.
263 • The psychosocial team (e.g. social worker, counsellor, psychologist).
264 • Your own faith groups and/or other support networks.

265   Ultimately, others in the team or outside the team such as healthcare chaplains or
266 spiritual leaders will be in apposition to provide you with clear guidance on spiritual
267 care matters. As mentioned, it is important to avoid making faith-related assump-
268 tions about the advice that can be provided. For example, assuming that a healthcare
269 chaplain of a single faith could not guide you on a care plan for a patient from a
270 different faith, or none, may prevent you from receiving important information and
271 advice. Healthcare chaplains, employed widely internationally, often operate on a
272 multifaith basis and will be either in a position to support the patient and family
273 directly or would have clear direction for support and contacts from other faiths (and
274 none). It is important to seek guidance from local or national policy in this regard.

275 ## 8.3   Documentation of Spiritual Care

276 The approach used for nursing and midwifery documentation varies across the
277 world. In some countries, nurses follow a systematic outline of written docu-
278 mentation built on systems such as the International Council of Nurses'

International Classification for Nursing Practice (ICNP) system [17] or the   279
NANDA-I (NANDA International, Incorporation) [18] and NIC (Nursing   280
Interventions Classification) [19]. These systems are used widely across the   281
USA, Portugal and Spain and provide not only ease of use for standardised   282
language within electronic healthcare systems but also a consistent nursing   283
focus. Within these systems, there is very often a category that guides the sup-   284
port and documentation of spiritual/existential/religious needs by nurses,   285
prompting them to outline the spiritual or other resources provided to patients   286
before evaluating and following-up. Although this area of the written docu-   287
mentation is not always consistently completed (for many reasons that are   288
beyond the scope of this chapter), they are a useful resource for nurses provid-   289
ing spiritual care to document spiritual care activity. For this reason, some of   290
our later examples in this chapter utilise these frameworks. In some other coun-   291
tries, the documentation of the spiritual assessment (Chap. 7) may be incorpo-   292
rated within the patient's care plan. At times, and we see this also in highly   293
specialised documentation systems that use the NANDA-I or ICNP in the   294
assessment of needs, resources and interventions are not documented. In some   295
cases, there is no history and culture in nursing/midwifery of spiritual assess-   296
ment, especially as it is a relatively novel area for nurses. In some cases, solely   297
documenting religion and/or referral to healthcare chaplaincy represents the   298
'intervention'. Regardless of whether or not the assessment and intervention of   299
spiritual care are clearly documented, it is good practice to document all care   300
given. Indeed, the premise of this chapter is that time should be taken to outline   301
the findings of the assessment and the specific interventions. The effects of   302
these should be later evaluated.   303

It is important to consider *why* and *how* we should document spiritual care.   304
In nursing and midwifery, we document conditions and aspects of care that are   305
vital for the patients' situations and important for follow-up. Spiritual care   306
documentation facilitates that the follow-up of patients becomes clear for   307
everyone working with the patient on an ongoing basis. Such documentation   308
become especially important where there are limited, or no verbal handover   309
practices, and each student/nurse/midwife may have to read the written reports   310
themselves to gain an update about each patient. If we do not document   311
patients' spiritual/existential/religious conditions, any knowledge about these   312
conditions risks not being transferred to other colleagues when the student/   313
nurse/midwife finishes their duty. Another important aspect is that documenta-   314
tion has a legal aspect. In case of a lawsuit, nursing documentation can be used   315
as a proof of what kind of care that was delivered or not delivered, and in the   316
case of no documentation, one cannot offer any defence of an action that was   317
not subsequently documented.   318

Documentation should be written so that the patient's integrity and confi-   319
dentiality are maintained, along with stating the intervention, and what needs   320
to be followed-up. In some healthcare systems, patients can log on and read the   321
documentation written by nurses and physicians immediately after they are   322
written. This should serve as a strong reminder for us to reflect on how to   323

324   balance the wording of our reports so that enough information is communi-
325   cated to the healthcare team to follow up on a patient's spiritual care, while
326   maintaining their integrity and confidentiality as appropriate.
327   We will now illustrate ways of how to complete nursing documentation in rela-
328   tion to spiritual care interventions. For each case we present, we will write about
329   different interventions and provide one example on how written nursing documen-
330   tation can be done.

331   8.4   Practice Examples to Exemplify Spiritual Care

332   In the following section, we will present four cases and discuss possible interven-
333   tions using Carson's [2] three main interventions: presence, the use of words and
334   taking actions. We will provide examples of how these interventions can be docu-
335   mented in some of the cases.

336   *8.4.1   Case 1: João*

> **Box 8.1: Case 1: João**
> *João is an 83-year-old man from Portugal, diagnosed 10 years ago with dementia. He lives with his wife, Maria. The couple visit the local church periodically. After their retirement, these church visits remain an important contact point where they meet friends and plan group trips for the summer. In the last year, João forgot his name and his wife's name too. There has been a functional decline, resulting in dependency. The multidisciplinary team told his wife that dementia means that brain cells are dying and that nothing can be done regarding memory stimulation. Maria is afraid to leave her husband alone—and in her words 'I am afraid to go outside as something might happen to my husband'. She cannot remember the last time she walked in the park or went to the local market. The local priest visits them regularly, and it surprises Maria that João can recite or respond to prayers during these visits and that when João prays, he can remember his name. When Maria asks him about his preferences, João frequently can tell what kind of food he would like to eat. However, during the health professionals' visit, João does not talk, does not answer questions and cannot even say what he thinks about or if he feels pain. João seems to feel good when looks at the painting they bought for the living room. Maria has placed it in the bedroom, in front of the bed.*

Below (Box 8.2) are some questions concerning the case study that may prompt   337
reflection and learning about this case. Take some time to consider the questions   338
before moving on in the chapter.   339

Box 8.2: Reflective Questions Regarding Case 1, João
1. What spiritual interventions do you suggest for João?
2. Do you consider ensuring privacy, helping people to connect, helping
    João to remember past experiences, listening to his or his wife's con-
    cerns, comforting and reassuring to be useful spiritual interventions
    for João?
3. How important is supporting João's and his wife's religious beliefs as
    a spiritual intervention?
4. What spiritual interventions can you suggest to support his wife to
    improve her capacity of care, help in dealing with difficult moments
    and preserve her quality of life?

Maria is very worried about João, since he is degrading in cognitive and func-   340
tional matter. One day he does not even know her, as he no longer knows the others.   341
In Portugal, nursing records are based on ICNP, and nurses' interventions on this   342
case are as follows: assess the degree of anxiety, monitor medication intake, pro-   343
mote adherence to the therapeutic regimen, monitor the presence of side effects of   344
the medication, monitoring confusion, managing communication, protecting the   345
person's integrity, cognitive stimulation, promoting distraction techniques and mon-   346
itoring sleep. João seems to respond very well to sensory interventions and when   347
involved in religious practices. However, the care plan is absent from nursing diag-   348
noses or specific interventions related to spirituality.   349

This case discloses the absence of spirituality in nursing records even when   350
nurses are aware of patients' preferences and rituals. Here we can find an opportu-   351
nity to use the foci, diagnoses, interventions and outcomes that are listed in interna-   352
tional classifications and effectively include in clinical records aiming to promote   353
comfort and dignity-preserving care.   354

8.4.2   Case 2: Jane   355

Box 8.3: Case 2: Jane
*Jane is a 36-year-old woman living in the Netherlands, who was involved in
an automobile accident 3 weeks ago. She was admitted to an Intensive Care
Unit (ICU). She is the mother of a 2-year-old girl and her husband does not
leave her side. Her condition is deteriorating. Since she is conscious and*

aware of her critical state, she shows increasing anxiety. She cries when the nurse come to check on her, crying out, 'please, tell me I'm not dying?' When nurses assessed Jane's value and belief systems, they found that the family had a strong faith, so when Jane became anxious and made this panicked comment about possible death they concluded and recorded in Jane's care plan that Jane showed 'spiritual distress' (diagnosis according to NANDA-I classification). As an intervention, they called in the reverend of Jane's faith community. However, the visits of the reverend seemed to have a counterproductive effect, as Jane was even more anxious after each visit. Jane did not want to talk about death and found no comfort in praying with the reverend and did seem at peace. The nurses did not fully understand how someone with a strong religious faith was so anxious of dying, although they understood her situation to be most difficult given her age, her young child and husband that she would leave behind should she die. To further support her, they initiated a more detailed spiritual assessment and discovered that it was not the dying itself that scared Jane but a feeling of leaving life 'unfinished'. It was the strong relationships with her husband and child that were about to be severed, which was a greater source of spiritual distress than the prospect of death. In her own words, 'How can I die, how can God let me die, when I feel so strongly that my life is not completed yet?'

356 Some questions about the case study that may prompt reflection and learning
357 about this case are given in Box 8.4. Take some time to consider the questions
358 before moving on in the chapter.

Box 8.4: Reflective Questions Regarding Case 2
1. Can you identify the professional qualities in the nurse that may have helped Jane as spiritual interventions?
2. What particular spiritual knowledge, skills and attitudes can the nurse draw upon to care for Jane and her husband?
3. Can you identify how *presence* as a spiritual intervention may have been useful for Jane and her husband?
4. Can you identify how *words* as a spiritual intervention may have been useful for Jane and her husband?
5. How would you write a report about Jane so other nurses could follow up?

This case demonstrated that an initial (informal) spiritual assessment (Chap. 7) needs to be followed up and documented at a later stage, and the results of each assessment should always be documented. This case also shows how important

nursing documentation and evaluation are to interpret whether or not interventions 359
worked. Evaluation is the only tool that will help to alter the care someone receives. 360
Therefore, Jane's anxiety would not have been remedied if the spiritual care were 361
not documented, or how Jane was reacting after the visits of the reverend. 362

Other spiritual interventions used were presence, words and specific actions. 363
Although it was not certain that Jane would die, the nurses knew that they had to 364
listen to Jane to learn how to help her in her spiritual questioning and help her 365
become less anxious. They intervened by listening and asking questions about what 366
is important to Jane and her family. They intervened by working in close collabora- 367
tion with Jane and her husband to develop a plan to activate the resources that gave 368
Jane the strength to face her critical situation. One intervention was the wish of Jane 369
to write the story of her life up until this point in time together with her husband. To 370
write her story could help her make sense of the event by fitting it into her life story 371
but also to pass it on to her daughter in the event she would die. The case also dem- 372
onstrates that sometimes interventions need to be creative. This approach echoes, 373
for example, the approach taken by Dr. Kate Piderman (a Healthcare Chaplain from 374
the Mayo Clinic in the USA), and the healthcare developed team, who developed 375
unique and innovative life stories with patients at end of life to understand their 376
legacy and share it with their family. 377

8.4.3 Case 3: Anna   378

Box 8.5: Case 3: Anna
*Anna is a 30-year-old woman living in Malta. At her 33rd week of her
first pregnancy, one afternoon she suddenly realised that her baby hadn't
moved all day. She had a job that kept her very busy, so she hadn't been
paying that much attention to her pregnancy for the last week. She had an
exceptionally active baby that seemed to move all the time. So, when
Anna didn't feel her move for a whole day, she got a sick, scared feeling
in her stomach. She called her midwife, Claire, who told Anna to come
over to hospital. When she reached the hospital, Claire explained that she
knew of cases when the mum did not feel movements and the baby was
still alive, so she told her not to worry. She quickly took her to the ultrasound department. Everyone encouraged Maria not to give up hope. Even
so, she felt really heavy. Michael, her husband, managed to come to the
hospital in time for the ultrasound. Anna cried and cried as she felt an
anguish and pain she had never felt before. In the room, there were two
persons wearing white coats looking at the screen as the scan proceeded.
Claire looked at the screen and then looked at the staff long and strong.
Everyone knew that the baby had died.*

379   Below are some questions about the case study that may prompt reflection and
380   learning about this case. Take some time to consider the questions before moving on
381   in the chapter.

> **Box 8.6: Reflective Questions Regarding Case 3**
>   1. What particular spiritual care competencies can the nurse draw upon
>   to care for Anna and her husband?
>   2. Can you identify how *presence* as spiritual interventions may have
>   been useful for Anna and her husband?
>   3. Can you identify how *words* as spiritual interventions may have been
>   useful for Anna and her husband?
>   4. What spiritual *interventions* can you suggest to support Anna and her
>   husband in dealing with these difficult moments?

382   Claire, the midwife, who stayed with Anna and Michael during the ultrasound
383   could see that the couple had a close relationship. Michael moved between support-
384   ing his wife and grieving himself. Claire decided to be with the parents in silence,
385   gently touching them on their shoulders, as a sign of understanding and presence,
386   but giving them time and space to comprehend the situation. Claire had experienced
387   such a situation before, so she started to plan how she best could prepare Anna and
388   Michael for what was ahead of them and how she could support them. After 20 min,
389   Claire asked how she could assist them in informing the family of what has hap-
390   pened and if they were ready to talk about the situation. Both Anna and Michael said
391   they wanted some information before they could talk to the family. Claire took them
392   to the room in the hospital where they could stay until the next phase of care (induced
393   delivery) was completed. In the room, Claire was conscious in relation to which
394   questions were asked by Anna and Michael as she tried to determine the limitations
395   of how much they could take in right now. She also carefully considered how ready
396   they were to think into the future, even the next days. She explained what to expect
397   next and that although the exact cause of death was uncertain at this point, this
398   would be investigated to provide further information. Claire, the midwife, knew that
399   an autopsy would be required but chose to hold this information from Anna and
400   Michael until a later point.
401   Anna moved in and out of despair, so Claire used time and gentle touch and tried
402   to follow the pace of the couple as she talked with them. After an hour, they felt
403   ready to call their parents and invite them to the hospital. Claire welcomed the fam-
404   ily and gave them some time and privacy to grieve together alone before she came
405   back into the room and was available for questions and to provide information. She
406   also brought refreshments, as it can be helpful to have something to hold on to such
407   as a cup of tea or coffee when you do not know what to say or do. Later on, in the
408   evening, Anna starts to ask questions: 'Why did this happen to us?' 'Have I done
409   something wrong?' Claire listens to her, and as there is not much she can say at the
410   moment, she confirms their pain and listens for any particular concerns. For

example, if Anna blames herself for doing or not doing. Claire managed to stay with   411
the couple without necessarily providing answers to give at the moment. Michael   412
was facilitated to sleep overnight at the hospital. Anna wore a crucifix. Claire won-   413
dered if the couple had a relationship to the church, and if there were resources, she   414
could use to support the couple and the family. This was an important observation   415
and explained how nurses and midwives need to be aware of subtle clues that indi-   416
cate spiritual needs. However, this was not the moment to investigate this as Anna   417
and Michael were absorbed in emotional and spiritual pain and grief.   418

At the end of the evening shift, Claire gave oral report to the nightshift and   419
recorded their grief, and her interventions in the nursing documentation: 420

> *Anna called me, her midwife, at 2pm today and told she was worried because she had not*   421
> *felt her child move all day. She was in her 33 weeks of pregnancy. Ultrasound showed that*   422
> *the child had died. Anna and her husband Michael are in deep grief. The extended family*   423
> *are informed and have visited them at the hospital this evening. Anna has started ask why*   424
> *this happened and if she has done something wrong. Her husband stays with her in the*   425
> *hospital tonight.*   426

This case clearly demonstrates the need for presence and kind words as spiritual   427
interventions and also the need for sensitive actions. Spiritual assessment needs to be   428
subtle as it was in this case and documented, so that later spiritual needs and resources   429
can be more rigorously assessed the following day to determine what rituals, sym-   430
bols and spiritual support might help with the acceptance of their baby's death.   431

8.4.4   Case 4: Carmen   432

Box 8.7: Case 4: Carmen
Carmen is a 63-year-old woman who lives in Spain. She attends primary care services for treatment of hypertension. She is married and has two adult children who do not live nearby. She usually has follow-up appointments with the nurse, David, every 2 months. For 3 months, her hypertension has been increasingly uncontrolled. During this time, she was showing little interest in her condition and behaving somewhat out of character. David suspected that she did was not adhering to treatment. On her last visit, he began to inquire about the reasons that led her to have this attitude. Carmen tells him that she feels very sad, she cries and has a hard time expressing herself. She says she is afraid of her situation because there are times when she is not able to control her crying and has even changed her healthy life habits, neglecting her illness, and her physical appearance. She stays at home and does not want to talk to anyone. She thinks her life is meaningless. She used to like going out with friends and helping others. She especially liked having time to talk with friends and family talking about her fears and getting mutual support, sometimes religious. She also liked being in touch with nature. She is much less inclined to do these things now.

433

> **Box 8.8: Reflective Questions Regarding Case 4**
> 1. What particular spiritual knowledge, skills and attitudes can the nurse draw upon to care for Carmen?
> 2. Can you identify how *presence* as a spiritual intervention may have been useful for Carmen?
> 3. Can you identify how *words* as a spiritual intervention may have been useful for Carmen?
> 4. What spiritual *interventions* can you suggest to support Carmen?

434 David was aware of Carmen's history of depression and asked about her current feel-
435 ings. David explores if she has had any spiritual support, what her beliefs are, and if she
436 practices any religion. Carmen, with her depressive symptomatology, says nothing.
437 David accepts the answer but is not totally convinced that he has fully addressed her
438 spiritual needs. Following a more thorough assessment and using the NANDA-I classi-
439 fication [18], he identifies that Carmen is at risk for spiritual distress and that the follow-
440 ing risk factors are presented: depression, loneliness and low self-esteem.

441 According to the NANDA-I and NIC, the following interventions should be
442 considered:

443 – Active listening.
444 – Advice.
445 – Spiritual support.

446 These interventions mirror the EPICC Spiritual Care Education Standard [7]
447 (Table 8.1), whereby communication and presence are key interventions with spe-
448 cific spiritual support. Specific interventions identified by David, relevant to
449 Carmen's situation, are outlined in Box 8.9.

> **Box 8.9: Examples of Key Spiritual Interventions Identified by David to Support Carmen in This Situation**
> • Display an awareness of and sensitivity to emotions.
> • Use silence/listening to encourage the expression of feelings, thoughts and concerns.
> • Determine the meaning of the message by reflecting on attitudes, past experiences and the current situation.
> • Avoid barriers to active listening (minimise feelings, offer simple solutions, do not interrupt, talk about yourself or end prematurely).
> • Encourage individuals to review their past life and focus on events and relationships that provided them with spiritual strength and support.
> • Encourage the use of spiritual resources, for example spiritual reading, if desired.
> • Refer to the spiritual advisor of individual's choice.

We observe how David is receptive of signs and symptoms as he listens to Carmen's story. He takes advantage of that information to be able to deepen his understanding of her situation. This case also reflects how the documentation is critical as records of subtle signs and changes in behaviour can be key considerations when planning appropriate interventions. This is especially important in areas such as primary health and many other areas where there is not a single named nurse looking after the patient and nursing staff vary over time. Documentation maintains continuity and allows for observation in changes in condition over time.

A useful element when using the NANDA-I taxonomy like this to guide nursing care is the clear need for follow-up evaluation with the patient. Evaluation of spiritual care is a component of the EPICC Spiritual Care Education Standard [7], and it means determining whether or not the actions and interventions had the intended outcome. Sometimes spirituality is an element of care that is overlooked (in terms of documentation) although nurses and midwives are encouraged to follow through on actions and interventions. In Carmen's case, and using the NANDA-I taxonomy, an evaluation will be carried out after a period of 1 month to assess whether the proposed actions have worked well. If Carmen's situation has not yet reached the aim set, but has evolved favourably, the timing of these interventions will be altered. In the event of a worsening, or the indicator remains at the same point, another therapeutic approach will need to be proposed.

8.5 Conclusion

This chapter follows on and builds on your learning from Chap. 7 where fundamental principles and practices with regard to spiritual assessment and the planning of spiritual care were outlined. Building on this, we introduced the concept of spiritual care intervention. We have outlined some guidance on how spiritual care interventions such as presence, words and actions may be used in clinical practice to support patients' and families' spiritual care. To support your understanding of these interventions, and how these might work in clinical practice, we have provided four practical case studies that we have explained and discussed within the text. This chapter has enabled you to become familiar with the fourth EPICC Spiritual Care Education Standard [7] competency related to spiritual care interventions and evaluation. It also facilitated sensitivity to patients' and families' spiritual needs and resources in various healthcare settings. Our aim has been to build your knowledge of spiritual interventions and to stimulate reflections on how to document and evaluate these.

8.6 Summary of the Main Points for Learning

The EPICC Spiritual Care Education Standard [7] competency related to spiritual care intervention and evaluation provides clear direction to nurses and midwives about planning spiritual care interventions.

Spiritual care attitudes might overlap with other important domains of nursing and midwifery practice, particularly in relation to interpersonal attitudes such as compassion, presence, empathy, openness, professional humility and trustworthiness.

Planning spiritual interventions must be individualised and patient-centred. Nurses and midwives need to be aware of their own limitations with spiritual care intervention and draw on expert resources when needed. Assumptive practices, discriminatory practices and proselytising should be avoided.

Documenting spiritual care is an important activity. Documentation methods vary internationally, and some resources are available, such as classifications and taxonomies (diagnoses, interventions and outcomes). Evaluation of spiritual care interventions, how spiritual needs have been met, and resources utilised is essential to ensure quality care. Ongoing reflection as a healthcare professional is an important aspect of spiritual care competency and in developing these skills.

References

1. Selman LE, et al. Patients' and Caregivers' needs, experiences, preferences and research priorities in spiritual care: a focus group study across nine countries. Palliat Med. 2018;32(1):216–30.
2. Carson VB. What is the essence of spiritual care? J Christ Nurs. 2011;28(3):173.
3. NHS Scotland. Spiritual care matters: an introductory resource for all NHS Scotland staff. 2010. https://www.nes.scot.nhs.uk/media/3723/spiritualcaremattersfinal.pdf.
4. Weathers E, McCarthy G, Coffey A. Concept analysis of spirituality: an evolutionary approach. Nurs Forum. 2016;51(2):79–96. https://doi.org/10.1111/nuf.12128.
5. Giske T, Cone P. Discerning the healing path—how nurses assist patients spiritually in diverse health care settings. J Clin Nurs. 2015;24(19–20):2926–35. https://doi.org/10.1111/jocn.12907.
6. Ross L, McSherry W, Giske T, van Leeuwen R, Schep-Akkerman A, Koslander T, Hall J, Steenfeldt VØ, Jarvis P. Nursing and midwifery students' perceptions of spirituality, spiritual care, and spiritual care competency: a prospective, longitudinal, correlational European study. Nurse Educ Today. 2018;67:64–71. https://doi.org/10.1016/j.nedt.2018.05.002.
7. Enhancing Nurses and Midwives' Competence in Providing Spiritual Care through Innovation, Education and Compassionate Care (EPICC). 2019. http://www.epicc-project.eu.
8. Papadopoulos I, Taylor G, Ali S, Aagard M, Akman O, Alpers LM, González-Gil T, et al. Exploring nurses' meaning and experiences of compassion: an international online survey involving 15 countries. J Transcult Nurs. 2017;28(3):286–95. https://doi.org/10.1177/1043659615624740.
9. Baart A. Theorie van de presentie ("theory of presence"). Utrecht: Lemma; 2004.
10. Bradfield Z, Duggan R, Hauck Y, Kelly M. Midwives being 'with woman': an integrative review. Women Birth. 2018;31(2):143–52. https://doi.org/10.1016/j.wombi.2017.07.011.
11. Koenig HG, King DE, Carson VB. Handbook in religion and health. New York: Oxford University Press; 2012.
12. RCN. Spirituality in nursing care: a pocket guide. London: The Royal College of Nursing; 2011.
13. Nightingale F. Notes on nursing: what it is, and what it is not, commemorative edn. London: Lippincott Williams and Wilkins; 1992.
14. Health Service Executive. Health services intercultural guide: responding to the needs of diverse religious communities and cultures in healthcare settings. 2009. http://www.hse.ie/ema/. Accessed 27 Jan 2020.

15. Health Service Executive. National Intercultural Health Strategy 2007–2012. Dublin: Health   534
    Service Executive; 2008.   535
16. College of Nurses of Ontario. Culturally Sensitive Care. 2009. https://rnao.ca/sites/rnao-ca/files/   536
    Embracing_Cultural_Diversity_in_Health_Care_-_Developing_Cultural_Competence.pdf.   537
17. International Council of Nurses' International Classification for Nursing Practice (ICNP)   538
    System. About ICNP. 2020. https://www.icn.ch/what-we-do/projects/ehealth-icnp/about-icnp.   539
    Accessed 17 Mar 2020.   540
18. Herdman TH, Kamitsuru S, editors. Nursing diagnoses: definitions & classification,   541
    2018–2020. 11th ed. New York, NY: Thieme; 2018.   542
19. Bulechek G, Butcher H, Dochterman J, Wagner C, editors. Nursing interventions classification   543
    (NIC). 6th ed. St. Louis, MO: Mosby; 2012.   544

Suggested Reading   545

Carson VB. What is the essence of spiritual care? J Christ Nurs. 2011;28(3):173.   546
Giske T, Cone P. Discerning the healing path—how nurses assist patients spiritually in diverse   547
    health care settings. J Clin Nurs. 2015;24(19–20):2926–35. https://doi.org/10.1111/jocn.12907.   548
RCN. Spirituality in nursing care: a pocket guide. London: The Royal College of Nursing; 2011.   549
Caldeira S, Timmins F. Implementing spiritual care interventions. Nurs Stand. 2017;31(34):54–60.   550
    https://doi.org/10.7748/ns.2017.e10313.   551

Chapter 9
Conclusions of the EPICC Journey and Future Directions

Adam Boughey, Wilfred McSherry, Linda Ross, Tove Giske, Josephine Attard, René van Leeuwen, and Tormod Kleiven

A. Boughey (✉)
Department of Nursing, School of Health and Social Care, Staffordshire University, Stoke-on-Trent, Staffordshire, England, UK
e-mail: adam.boughey@staffs.ac.uk

W. McSherry
Department of Nursing, School of Health and Social Care , Staffordshire University, University Hospitals of North Midlands NHS Trust,
Stoke-on-Trent, Staffordshire, England, UK

VID University College, Bergen/Oslo, Norway
e-mail: w.mcsherry@staffs.ac.uk

L. Ross
Faculty of Life Sciences and Education, School of Care Sciences, University of South Wales, Pontypridd, UK
e-mail: linda.ross@southwales.ac.uk

T. Giske
Faculty of Health Studies, VID Specialized University, Bergen, Norway
e-mail: tove.giske@vid.no

J. Attard
University of Malta, Msida, Malta
e-mail: josephine.attard@um.edu.mt

R. van Leeuwen
Viaa Christian University of Applied Sciences, Zwolle, The Netherlands
e-mail: r.vanleeuwen@viaa.nl

T. Kleiven
VID Specialized University, Stavanger, Norway
e-mail: tormod.kleiven@vid.no

© Springer Nature Switzerland AG 2021
W. McSherry et al. (eds.), *Enhancing Nurses' and Midwives' Competence in Providing Spiritual Care*, https://doi.org/10.1007/978-3-030-65888-5_9

> **Learning Objectives**
> This chapter will enable you to:
>
> 1. Understand the structure of the EPICC project according to its intellectual outputs and how these were achieved through a variety of specific project events.
> 2. Reflect on the ways in which the EPICC project was innovative in meeting its ambitious aims and objectives, particularly in supporting collaborations between many stakeholders from different countries.
> 3. Explore how the EPICC project may advance and support the development of spiritual care education in the future.

9.1 Introduction

To appreciate the context of the EPICC project and the unique contribution each previous chapter of this text has made to outline important components of EPICC, it is worth recapping on why the project was needed, and how this has informed key developments in spirituality and spiritual care in nursing and midwifery. As detailed in the introduction, the EPICC project has represented, in many respects, the cumulation of several decades of pioneering and seminal research for the contributors of this text. Many contributors have dedicated much of their career, and most of their research time over the 3 years of the EPICC project to *enhancing nurses' and midwives' competence in providing spiritual care through innovative education and compassionate care* (EPICC). This acronym is therefore fitting, in terms of both representing this pioneering work and, akin to its similar term 'epic', representing an ambitious and significant attempt to promote excellence in spiritual care education in nursing and midwifery by aspiring for standardisation in the teaching of these concepts.

We believe, and have confidence that you do also, that upholding spirituality and spiritual care in nursing and midwifery are important in ensuring that each person receives healthcare that is person-centred and holistic. However, there is often disconnection between professional regulators' aspirations for high-quality spiritual care and actual practice. For example, in the United Kingdom, the Nursing and Midwifery Council (NMC) in their standards of competence for registered nurses [1] highlights that all nurses have a duty of care to assess, 'physical, social, cultural, psychological, spiritual, genetic and environmental factors' (p. 8). Assessment of these needs was also highlighted in the latest NMC [2] Future Nurse standards where 'registered nurses need to prioritise the needs of people when assessing and reviewing their mental, physical, cognitive, behavioural, social and spiritual needs' (p. 13). A key attribute of these professional nursing standards is that they pertain to the assessment of patients' needs. However, there is surprisingly little mention of the importance of spiritual *care*, although the notion of holistic care is mentioned. In contrast, the NMC standards of proficiency for midwives [3] does have more specific reference to spirituality and

spiritual care, by referring to how, 'midwives optimise normal physiological pro-   36
cesses, and support safe physical, psychological, social, cultural and spiritual situ-   37
ations' (p. 4). In this respect, spiritual care is considered from the perspective of,   38
'spiritual *safety* of the woman and their newborn infants' (p. 10), and the links   39
between spiritual care and 'the woman's, father's/partner's, and family's wishes   40
and *religious/spiritual beliefs and faith*' (p. 50). Despite these regulatory stan-   41
dards for nursing and midwifery, there is evidence of failure to meet spiritual   42
needs in the provision of healthcare. For example, barriers to implementing spiri-   43
tual care include: challenges in defining what 'spirituality' means; what the role   44
of the nurse (or midwife) is in the provision of spiritual care; having sufficient   45
time in busy healthcare environments to be with, listen to and engage with patients;   46
and having sufficient training and education in spiritual care [4].   47

It is the latter point of professional education in spiritual care that has been the   48
core focus of the EPICC project. In a review of research into spiritual care in nurs-   49
ing, Ross [5] highlighted that a lack of educational preparedness in spiritual care in   50
nursing has been evident for approximately 30 years. Specifically, Narayanasamy   51
[6] highlighted how nurses felt under-prepared to provide spiritual care and that   52
spiritual care education was lacking in preregistration nursing curricula [7]. Within   53
Ross's review [5], there was a mention of research outlining the testing of various   54
spiritual care competencies [8]. The clear message of the review was that there   55
needed to be more coordination and systematisation of research into spirituality and   56
spiritual care education. A further review by Cockell and McSherry [9] of spiritual   57
care in nursing further highlighted the developing focus and importance of effective   58
spiritual care education. Specifically, that educational preparedness helps to reduce   59
nurses' perceptions of insecurity in providing spiritual care [10] and that the impact   60
of ensuring spiritual care education is incorporated within preregistration curricula   61
help nurses to further understand the notion of holistic care. Furthermore, at the   62
time, there was development of a measure (the Spiritual Care Competence Scale   63
[SCCS]) to assess the spiritual care competence of nurses [11, 12].   64

Assessing spiritual care competence in nursing and midwifery was fast becom-   65
ing an important issue to address the lack of preregistration educational preparation   66
in spirituality and spiritual care. This led to the development and implementation of   67
two major studies that would become the empirical foundation for the EPICC proj-   68
ect. The first (pilot) study undertook a cross-sectional, multinational pilot study in   69
Europe to assess undergraduate nurses'/midwives' perceptions of spirituality/spiri-   70
tual care, along with their perceived competence in delivering spiritual care [13].   71
Ross et al. [14] then explored the factors contributing to undergraduate nurses'/   72
midwives' perceived competence in providing spiritual care. The second (main)   73
study with a larger sample of initially 2193 undergraduate nursing/midwifery stu-   74
dents across 21 universities in eight countries explored perceptions of spirituality/   75
spiritual care over time, along with competence and the factors contributing to the   76
development of spiritual care competency [15].   77

In the light of the above studies, two questions that remained was how nursing/   78
midwifery educators could (1) be supported to enhance the spiritual care compe-   79
tency of students who do not identify as religious and (2) encourage students   80

81 holding a narrow view of spirituality/spiritual care to broaden their perspective to be
82 inclusive of all faith and no faith backgrounds. This provided the foundation for the
83 EPICC project.

84 ## 9.2   Innovation

85 From the outset of the project, the EPICC Strategic Partners ensured that the project
86 responded to the voice of students, nurses and midwives; mindful of transnational
87 research indicating that nurses and midwives require more educational preparation
88 to address patients' spiritual needs [13–18]. It was a priority for the project to
89 remain action-oriented and produce resources that would be of practical value to
90 nursing/midwifery education across Europe and internationally. This ambition
91 required an action learning cycles [19] methodology and co-production between all
92 project stakeholders, as illustrated in Chap. 1 through the 'EPICC triangle'. For one
93 side of the triangle: the EPICC Strategic Partners—already acclaimed experts in
94 spirituality and spiritual care—it was crucial to ensure that the other two sides of the
95 triangle, comprising EPICC Participants (within Europe) and EPICC Participants+
96 (within Europe and internationally) co-produced the project's resources. The trans-
97 national aspect of the EPICC project represented a significant innovation, by involv-
98 ing EPICC Participants from 21 European countries and Participants+ from Europe
99 and three countries from outside of Europe. Indeed, the six EPICC Strategic Partners
100 represented an alliance from five European countries, and a formalisation of the
101 previous European Spirituality Research Network for Nursing and Midwifery, as
102 outlined in Chap. 1.
103   These cross-cultural partnerships were particularly important, as the authors are
104 not aware of any previous projects that have addressed spirituality and spiritual care
105 in nursing/midwifery education with the level of regional and international engage-
106 ment as seen in EPICC. The partnerships, collaborations and stakeholders' engage-
107 ment were a considerable strength of the project and helped to ensure innovation by
108 involving stakeholders at every stage, in particular when co-producing the various
109 project outputs (outlined below). The partnerships of nursing/midwifery and other
110 professions from a range of diverse geopolitical regions across Europe has resulted
111 in being able to capture the cultural, religious and ethnic diversity that exists in
112 Europe. This has helped to provide assurance that nurses and midwives, when
113 assessed as competent in meeting the requirements outlined in the EPICC Standard
114 for Spiritual Care Education (outlined below), will be able to relate positively and
115 sensitively to patients'/clients' spirituality and spiritual care across a wide range of
116 European contexts. By inspiring generations of nurses and midwives in spirituality
117 and spiritual care through the work of EPICC, it is hoped that future nurses and
118 midwives will be educated and supported as to the diversity of opinion and belief
119 that exists with regard to understanding spirituality and spiritual care, not just in
120 Europe, but internationally.

9.3 Intellectual Outputs and Development of Project Resources

As mentioned in Chap. 1, the EPICC project comprised three intellectual outputs (O), which Erasmus+ [20] considers to be activities 'that results in tangible and meaningful outcomes, such as publications and course materials'. The three intellectual outputs included:

1. Establishment and promoting stakeholder engagement (O1).
2. Development and refinement of key project resources (O2).
3. Sharing of best practice in spiritual care education and launch of an on-going EPICC Network (O3).

9.3.1 Output 1

EPICC stakeholders' engagement was crucial to achieve O1, and the EPICC Project Manager (Dr. Adam J. Boughey) oversaw the daily management of the project and initial contact with potential Participants and Participants+. O1 was achieved through two 'Multiplier Events' (ME), which were 'organised to share the intellectual output of a project with a wider audience' [20]. Careful planning, delivery and evaluation of these events ensured that stakeholder engagement and collaboration could be promoted (ME 1) and that the long-term sustainability of the EPICC partnership could be strengthened and maintained (ME 2).

The first project event, ME 1, was hosted by Staffordshire University (UK) in April 2017 and established the project's foundation by preparing stakeholders (the three groups of the EPICC triangle) regarding the intellectual outputs and project activities. The purpose of ME 1 was to bring together as many Participants and Participants+ as possible, increasing awareness of the project and strategic partnership across Europe to ensure a unique branding and identity. Three objectives of ME 1 were planned to:

1. Present findings from the multinational studies[1] of student nurses'/midwives' spiritual care competencies and identify implications for nursing/midwifery education, practice and the project.
2. Identify strategies to ensure the significant findings from the studies were shared and adopted by nursing and midwifery from within the EPICC Strategic Partners' and EPICC Participants' institutions and countries.
3. Explore how the findings from the study could be disseminated to inform nursing/midwifery education and practice, locally within EPICC Strategic Partners' and EPICC Participants' curricula, and more broadly within Europe and internationally.

---

[1] Ross et al. [13–15].

Table 9.1 Multiplier event 1	t1.1
Day 1	t1.2
Keynotes	t1.3
1. Opening and welcome	t1.4
2. What is the EPICC project: Relevance to nursing and midwifery practice and education?	t1.5
Poster displays and networking	t1.6
Workshops	t1.7
1. Review/discuss transnational studies' findings:	t1.8
• What do the findings mean for equipping undergraduate nurses/midwives (university/	t1.9
practice) for providing spiritual care?	t1.10
• Challenges/opportunities?	t1.11
2. Synthesise a shared understanding of 'best practice' in spiritual care education	t1.12
3. Action planning	t1.13
4. Feedback	t1.14
Summary of main findings and conclusions	t1.15
Day 2	t1.16
Keynotes	t1.17
1. What do we mean by competence in spiritual care? Developing the Spiritual Care	t1.18
Competence Scale	t1.19
2. Nurses' and midwives' acquisition of competency in spiritual care: A focus on education	t1.20
3. The impact of pre-registration nurses' spirituality education on clinical practice: A	t1.21
grounded theory investigation	t1.22
Poster displays and networking	t1.23
Workshops	t1.24
1. Share tips/experiences of how you have equipped students for giving spiritual care	t1.25
2. Moving forward:	t1.26
• Mapping exercise for benchmarking local audits of current practice	t1.27
• Agree means of continued engagement/communication	t1.28
• Role of the EPICC project website	t1.29

To ensure equality and diversity in the recruitment of Participants and Participants+, efforts were made to engage nursing/midwifery educators from across Europe, and stakeholders across Europe and internationally via email, social media and the EPICC website (www.epicc-network.org). The aim was to generate awareness and interest and invite the Participants and Participants+ to ME 1 to meet each other, the Strategic Partners, Project Manager, and the project support team. Ensuring early contact with nursing/midwifery educators and stakeholders created a 'snowball' effect as such, where word of the project spread between influencers with an interest in the study of spirituality and spiritual care, thus supporting recruitment.

Keynote lectures highlighted the project's relevance to nursing/midwifery education, key findings from the transnational studies, what is considered to be competence in spiritual care, and the impact of spiritual care education on clinical practice (Table 9.1). Over two intense days, stakeholders reviewed significant findings from

the transnational studies and how findings inform the development of nursing/mid-   170
wifery education and practice. These small groups of stakeholders thrived on eclec-   171
tic, respectful and constructive discussions of the facilitators and inhibitors of   172
spiritual care practice. These sessions of innovative educational approaches were   173
captured by means of PowerPoint presentations and posters. Later into ME 1, stake-   174
holders synthesised a common understanding of 'best practice' in spiritual care edu-   175
cation based on the previous discussions, which enabled Participants to return to   176
their higher education institutions and undertake any innovative curriculum devel-   177
opment to develop the focus on spiritual care education in nursing/midwifery.   178

   ME 1 workshop discussions indicated that the findings from the transnational   179
studies were optimistic and welcomed. Despite complexity in defining spirituality   180
and spiritual care, it was accepted that spiritual care concerns the 'small things' that   181
'mean a lot' to patients/clients. Spiritual care was considered to manifest in a variety   182
of forms, and it was important that the clinician is receptive to the dimension of   183
spirituality, by actively listening and acknowledging the existence and presence of   184
another person (human 'being'). Discussions focused on the need for greater inte-   185
gration of spirituality/spiritual care in the bio-psycho-social model or biomedical   186
model of healthcare provision. It was also highlighted that spiritual care was consid-   187
ered to be too-often focused on the provision of care and support at the end of life,   188
and not focused enough on the provision of care and support throughout the lifespan.   189

   Group discussions also focused on perceived competence in spiritual care and a   190
student's possible disparity before and after exposure to clinical practice. Generally,   191
there was consensus of the importance of ensuring that spirituality/spiritual care   192
remains an educational and professional development priority for all clinicians. Of   193
particular mention was that Healthcare Support Workers (HCSWs) were considered   194
an important group to focus on in terms of providing education and training con-   195
cerning the provision of spiritual care, due to the significant time they have with   196
patients/clients. There was critical discussion concerning the notion of whether it is   197
necessary to provide education and training concerning spiritual care, if spirituality   198
is something that is 'innate' to all humans. However, this was considered an area   199
that requires some level of 'formalisation' in terms of education and its focus in on-   200
going personal and professional development in nursing and midwifery; indeed,   201
that it is the responsibility of every clinician to support students and other staff in   202
providing spiritual care. Despite this, discussions indicated practical challenges   203
when providing spiritual care due to the workplace/workforce culture, 'taking time'   204
to be with patients/clients in the face of other pressures, and with 'spiritual care'   205
perhaps seen to be 'someone else's' job or the preserve of the chaplain/priest, etc.   206

   ME 2 was the fourth (and final) project event in July 2019, hosted by the   207
University of South Wales (UK) and aimed to showcase and disseminate the find-   208
ings from the entire project and to formally establish and launch the EPICC Network.   209
To meet this ambitious task in capturing the essence, but also highlight the complex-   210
ity of the project's achievements, three objectives of ME 2 were planned to: 211

212 1. Provide case studies and experiences from the EPICC Strategic Partners and
213   EPICC Participants in the form of 'ViPER'[2] sessions (10-min presentations,
214   10-min moderated discussion).
215 2. Share lessons learned and develop good practice by highlighting the facilitators
216   and inhibitors in the provision of spiritual care in nursing/midwifery, through
217   ViPER and EPICC Adoption Toolkit 'taster' sessions.
218 3. Capture experiences of Participants in how they utilised the EPICC Gold
219   Standard Matrix for Spiritual Care Education, the EPICC Standard, and the
220   teaching/learning strategies from the EPICC Adoption Toolkit.

221   To ensure that ME 2 succeeded in showcasing and disseminating project outputs,
222 involvement from stakeholders was key. Participants and Participants+ were informed
223 of the event at the outset of the project and throughout each of the other project events
224 (Learning/Teaching/Training Activities). Having a website as a central project 'hub' to
225 share information and provide open access to project resources was a high priority from
226 the outset. By the time of ME 2, the project website had significantly evolved from its
227 humble beginnings at ME 1, due to the work of the Project Manager and Mr. Tom Ward
228 (Project and Portfolio Coordinator, Staffordshire University). Along with the website
229 development, there was extensive liaison with the Marketing and Communications
230 Team and the Brand Officer (Mr. Tim Deville, Staffordshire University) to work on the
231 development of a unique colour palette and new project logos that would become the
232 foundation for the launch of the EPICC Network at ME 2. These branding develop-
233 ments were an important milestone in the public appearance of the project and how the
234 EPICC Network would evolve as a familiar, but also distinctive, entity for future stake-
235 holder collaboration. The new project branding and website development also provided
236 the foundation by which all project outputs (resources and learning materials) could be
237 collated and disseminated with ease to ensure free and open access to all stakeholders
238 and others outside of the project interested in the subject matter.
239   During ME 2, over a course of two intense days (Tables 9.2 and 9.3), there was a
240 combination of keynote lectures to help consolidate the importance and significance of
241 the achievements of the project and how this implicates nursing/midwifery education
242 and practice. Further lectures by the Strategic Partners and Project Manager provided
243 delegates with an overview of the project's journey, along with how the key resources
244 and outputs had developed. At this stage of the project it was important that stakeholders
245 had a clear understanding of the bigger picture of the processes and outcomes and the
246 significance of the intense work that had been undertaken over the previous 3 years. It
247 was anticipated that ME 2, being the final project event, would help to consolidate stake-
248 holders' resolution to enhance nurses' and midwives' competence in providing spiritual
249 care through innovative education and compassionate care.
250   It was important for stakeholders to understand how two key outputs of O2
251 (explained below): (1) the EPICC Standard for Spiritual Care Education, and (2) the
252 Gold Standard Matrix for Spiritual Care Education provided a foundation to develop

---

[2]ViPER: Visual Presentation with Expert Review [21] represents the delivery of research presentations to promote networking by generating interaction and discussion, rather than a typical didactic
approach.

Table 9.2 Multiplier event 2   t2.1

Day 1	t2.2

Keynotes   t2.3
1. Opening and welcome   t2.4
2. Humanising care: What is it to attend to the whole person?   t2.5
3. Why providing spiritual care is important: A personal perspective   t2.6

Poster displays and networking   t2.7

Keynotes   t2.8
1. The EPICC Journey: Overview of the EPICC Project and its outputs. The big picture   t2.9
2. Showcasing the EPICC Adoption Toolkit   t2.10

Showcasing the EPICC Standard and Matrix: Snapshots from across Europe   t2.11
ViPER sessions (10-min presentations, 10-min moderated discussion)   t2.12

Launch and showcasing of the EPICC website   t2.13

Conclusion and quiet reflection   t2.14

Inaugural professorial lecture   t2.15
The changing landscape of spirituality in healthcare: Time travel across three decades   t2.16

Table 9.3 Multiplier event 2   t3.1

Day 2	t3.2

Short stories: Spiritual care making a difference or not   t3.3
- Clinical psychology: Spirituality in the context of older people's mental health   t3.4
- Clinical nursing: Making a difference to a stroke patient's care   t3.5
- Student nursing: Trying out an example from the EPICC Adoption Toolkit in practice   t3.6
- Patient's story: Scared of dying   t3.7
- Carer's story: Nurses who can see into your soul   t3.8
- Quiet reflection   t3.9

Next steps   t3.10
- Evaluation of the EPICC project   t3.11
- EPICC Network and International Student Conference (30/09/20 to 02/10/20)   t3.12

ViPER Poster displays and networking   t3.13

EPICC Adoption Toolkit 'taster' sessions (20 min)   t3.14

Competencies 2, 3: Taking a spiritual history	Competency 1: Life Tree	Competency 2: Recognising spiritual needs	Competency 2: Handy conversations	t3.15 t3.16 t3.17
Competency 1: Faith history	Competencies 1, 2: Introduction to the Diamond Model	Competency 4: Documentation	Competencies 3, 4: Link nurse @ spiritual care	t3.18 t3.19 t3.20

Role play (competencies 2 and 3)   t3.21
- Cardiac arrest: 'Am I going to die, nurse?'   t3.22
- Spiritual care at end of life   t3.23
- Student opportunity to accompany service users to Lourdes   t3.24

ViPER Poster displays and networking   t3.25

Keynote   t3.26
'How to treat people'   t3.27
- Conclusion and evaluation   t3.28
- Quiet reflection   t3.29

253   innovative approaches for preregistration nursing/midwifery education. The imple-
254   mentation of these outputs by Participants/Participants+ across Europe were show-
255   cased through visual presentations with expert review (ViPER) on day one. These
256   sessions were supplemented with EPICC Adoption Toolkit 'taster' sessions on day
257   two, showcasing how stakeholders had designed, implemented, and evaluated educa-
258   tional strategies (teaching sessions). Prior to ME 2, stakeholders emailed their educa-
259   tional strategies to the Project Manager, who collated them into a standardised format,
260   thus forming the EPICC Adoption Toolkit as an open resource on the project website.
261   Standardisation ensured that educational strategies had clear and consistent informa-
262   tion, such as author(s), mapping to one or more of the EPICC Standard competencies,
263   focus on nursing/midwifery, etc., learning objectives, educators' roles, resources,
264   assessment and references.

265   An innovative aspect of ME 2 was the incorporation of activities, providing
266   stakeholders with opportunities to self-reflect, network, and attend 'self-care' ses-
267   sions. 'Self-care' was important to address as developing self-awareness and con-
268   nection beyond the self are important in the provision of spiritual care [22].
269   Stakeholders were invited to an inaugural professorial lecture by Strategic Partner,
270   Professor Linda Ross. This lecture offered a professional overview of how spiritual-
271   ity and spiritual care has changed since the 1980s/1990s.

272   *9.3.2   Output 2 and 3*

273   The success with O1 depended on the strength of partnerships, collaborations and
274   stakeholder engagement and provided a foundation for the successes with O2 and
275   O3. Although O2 and O3 were distinct, with O2 focusing on development and
276   refinement of project resources and O3 sharing best practice and launching the
277   EPICC Network, O2 and O3 events were conceptually similar. Two Learning/
278   Teaching/Training Activity (LTTA) events—one for each intellectual output (2 and
279   3)—enabled the development, refinement, and dissemination of the three project
280   resources. These were: (1) the EPICC Gold Standard Matrix for Spiritual Care
281   Education, (2) the EPICC Standard for Spiritual Care Education, and (3) the EPICC
282   Adoption Toolkit. Although outlined above in O1 for the ME 2 activities, key
283   aspects of their development, refinement and dissemination will be outlined here for
284   O2 and O3. Both LTTA events lasted 5 days each and comprised intensive small
285   group and plenary discussions to achieve consensus regarding the project resources.
286   Further details of the consensus procedure between June 2017 and February 2019
287   can be found in van Leeuwen et al. [23].

288   LTTA 1 was the second project event in October 2017, hosted by Viaa: Christian
289   University of Applied Sciences (Zwolle, Netherlands), and aimed to inform the on-
290   going development of a draft EPICC Standard, Matrix, and Adoption Toolkit. The
291   objectives of LTTA 1 were to:

292   1. Enhance the cultural sensitivity regarding spirituality and spiritual care.
293   2. Define the key nursing and midwifery competencies in spiritual care.

3. Review effective educational practices (learning objectives, activities, outcomes and assessment) in relation to spiritual care.

4. Clarify the conditions regarding the implementation and testing of an educational matrix in education practice.

LTTA 1 developed EPICC stakeholders' awareness of the intense work that was required to:

1. Continue promoting stakeholder engagement and collaborations following Multiplier Event 1.
2. Collaborate to define and reach consensus of the key nursing/midwifery spiritual care competences, which were to become the basis of the draft EPICC Standard.
3. Share diverse educational practices and strategies to promote spiritual care education, which were to become the basis of the draft EPICC Adoption Toolkit.
4. Consider how the draft EPICC Standard and Adoption Toolkit resources are situated more broadly within the cultural, social and political environment in which spiritual care competency develops; represented by the EPICC Matrix.

As seen in Table 9.4, LTTA 1 was a significant process for the project in having provided stakeholders with opportunities for discussions and reflection to develop resources. Over five intense days, stakeholders contributed significant knowledge

Table 9.4 Learning/Teaching/Training Activity 1

Day 1
Activities
Plenary (spiritual care education):
1. Where do we come from, and where are we now? Presentation of the results of the Multiplier Event 1
2. Competences, outcomes, strategies and assessment. Results from an online survey amongst EPICC participants
Teaching and learning:
1. Reflection on educational strategies and learning outcomes (expert perspectives)
(a). Patients
(b). Professionals
(c). Educationalists
Poster displays (learning outcomes) and networking

Days 2–5		
Activities	Focus	Day
Teaching and learning, and plenary learning sessions, followed with presentation and synthesis of learning outcomes from the group sessions (reflections, discussions and conclusions)	• Spiritual care competencies as the foundation for spiritual care education	2
	• Effective teaching in spiritual care	3
	• Introduction in assessment of spiritual care education	4
	• Implementation and evaluation of EPICC Standard and Matrix	5
	• Evaluation/reflections on LTTA 1	

312 and experience of spiritual care education. During the event, many were situated in
313 the same location where LTTA 1 took place. This resulted in opportunities outside
314 of the event itinerary for networking and sharing knowledge, skills, and experiences
315 in spirituality and spiritual care. LTTA 1 also offered stakeholders with unique
316 opportunities for an excursion to the Ethics Simulation Laboratory (Viaa University).
317   The first draft of the EPICC Standard was the key resource developed during
318 LTTA 1. What was particularly innovative about the development of the EPICC
319 Standard was how its development was based on the pioneering work by Dr.
320 Josephine Attard (Maltese Strategic Partner), who for her PhD developed the first
321 spiritual care competency framework for pre-registration nursing and midwifery
322 education with seven domains and 51 items [24, 25]. During the first part of LTTA
323 1, analysis of EPICC stakeholders' survey responses of agreement or disagreement
324 to the 51 items of Dr. Attard's competency framework was presented to further
325 inform the development and refinement of the EPICC Standard.
326   As detailed in van Leeuwen et al. [23], an online survey was completed by 35
327 EPICC stakeholders from 18 European countries prior to the LTTA 1, where they
328 were invited to indicate their agreement or disagreement (5-point Likert scale) with
329 each item across the seven domains. Most respondents (25) were affiliated with
330 nursing; two respondents with midwifery; and eight respondents with bioethics,
331 philosophy, theology, social work, clinical psychology, research and teaching. Most
332 were involved with undergraduate and/or postgraduate education, or research con-
333 cerning spiritual needs, spiritual care education and holistic well-being. During
334 LTTA 1, stakeholders engaged in a continuous process of discussion and voting on
335 how to merge survey items and domains into a more compact standard that could be
336 easier to comprehend. This consensus procedure was aided by attending to the cog-
337 nitive, functional and behavioural (knowledge, skills and attitudes) aspects of spiri-
338 tual care competency. These aspects enabled significantly more refinement of the
339 various spiritual care competencies, whilst ensuring that (1) the complexity of each
340 item and their conceptual focus were retained and (2) the EPICC Standard was not
341 overwhelmingly complex to be of practical use. It was this nine-competency draft
342 EPICC Standard that Participants implemented and tested at their respective univer-
343 sities/institutions/organisations before LTTA 2 that was a key success of LTTA 1
344 and provided a strong foundation for LTTA 2.
345   LTTA 2 was the third project event in September 2018, hosted by the University
346 of Malta (Valletta, Republic of Malta), and aimed to review the testing and imple-
347 mentation of the draft EPICC Standard, Matrix, and Adoption Toolkit. The objec-
348 tives of LTTA 2 were to:

349 1. Review Participants' experiences from using the EPICC Standard in their respec-
350   tive universities/institutions/organisations and capture feedback from
351   Participants+ (project stakeholders) regarding the EPICC Standard.
352 2. Capture the cultural, spiritual and religious impact of the EPICC Standard, by
353   identifying facilitators and inhibitors.
354 3. Refine the EPICC Standard and further development of the EPICC Matrix, ahead
355   of the final project event (ME 2).

As seen in Table 9.5, LTTA 2 continued the development and refinement of the   356
project resources (EPICC Standard, Matrix and Adoption Toolkit) following LTTA   357
1. A similar format to LTTA 1 of in-depth discussions and reflective learning was   358
chosen over five intense days for LTTA 2. The event was also graced with atten-   359
dance from high profile speakers, external to the project, including Maltese govern-   360
ment ministers and senior religious officials.   361

By the time of LTTA 2, the project was well underway, and stakeholders had   362
plenty of contact with each other in respect of implementing and testing the draft   363
EPICC Standard and Matrix. LTTA 2 was successful in providing Participants with   364
important opportunities in reporting on how they used the EPICC Standard and   365
Matrix. In the run-up to LTTA 2, Participants were allocated a 'mentor' (one of the   366
Strategic Partners) to support them in their implementation and testing of the draft   367
EPICC Standard (and Matrix). The value of these resources was evident from all   368
Participants who provided an overview of their testing and implementation in LTTA   369

Table 9.5 Learning/Teaching/Training Activity 2	t5.1
Day 1	t5.2
Activities	t5.3
1. Welcome and introduction to the event	t5.4
2. Evaluations of the draft EPICC Standard (Participant presentations 1)	t5.5
Day 2	t5.6
Activities	t5.7
1. Evaluations of the draft EPICC Standard (Participant presentations 2)	t5.8
2. Draft EPICC Standard and Matrix workshops (strengths, weaknesses, opportunities,	t5.9
strengths)	t5.10
Day 3	t5.11
The cultural, spiritual/religious impact of the EPICC Standard and Matrix: Forum	t5.12
1. Welcome	t5.13
2. Keynote 1 (Director of Nursing)	t5.14
3. Keynote 2 (Parliamentary Secretary)	t5.15
4. Forum discussion (EPICC stakeholders)	t5.16
5. Spiritual care in secular midwifery: The Danish case	t5.17
6. The impact of spiritual care standards in nursing: Two examples from the Netherlands	t5.18
7. Mental health and policy (EPICC: A view from Wales and from the Royal College of	t5.19
Nursing, UK)	t5.20
Tribute to the late, Professor Donia Baldacchino, former Maltese Strategic Partner	t5.21
Day 4	t5.22
Refinements of the draft EPICC Standard, Matrix, and Adoption Toolkit	t5.23
Discussion: Finalisation of the terminology	t5.24
Refinements to the draft EPICC Standard and Matrix	t5.25
Refinements to the draft EPICC Adoption Toolkit	t5.26
Development of the International EPICC Network for Spiritual Care in Nursing and	t5.27
Midwifery	t5.28
Students' Conference	t5.29
Day 5	t5.30
• Evaluation of LTTA 2	t5.31
• From Malta to Wales: Participants' input to ME 2	t5.32

370   2. This assured Strategic Partners of the value in having focused on the development
371   of these resources at LTTA 1 and provided a foundation by which these resources
372   would undergo refinement in LTTA 2. Ultimately, the promotion of nurses' and
373   midwives' competence in spiritual care education remained central to the refine-
374   ment process.
375   Participants' presentations indicated the extensive work that was undertaken to
376   map the nine draft EPICC Standard competencies against existing nursing/mid-
377   wifery curricula. It was clear that in many instances, there was already considerable
378   overlap in the key elements of the EPICC Standard and what was already been
379   taught. Typically, this was in modules such as professional, legal and ethical consid-
380   erations; introductory theology; philosophy; cultural studies; communication; lead-
381   ership and management; dignity and empowerment; and compassionate and
382   person-centred care. Because of the transnational project, resources such as the
383   EPICC Standard required translation into national languages, such as Croatian,
384   Flemish and Polish, and this work was on-going at the point of LTTA 2. Due to the
385   conceptual complexities of spirituality and how spiritual care is understood in a
386   variety of increasingly secular societies across Europe, it was clear that aspects of
387   the EPICC Standard and Matrix would require adaptation to the local nursing/mid-
388   wifery educational context and clinical practice. Notwithstanding these complexi-
389   ties, it was clear that the testing and implementation of project resources had
390   prompted a range of curricula reviews and developments; and had encouraged addi-
391   tional research and development in spirituality and spiritual care at Participants'
392   institutions. In this respect, the project demonstrated innovation in how it brought
393   together many stakeholders from different countries, each with their own geopoliti-
394   cal, cultural and educational differences.
395   With the foundation of Participants' testing and implementation of the EPICC
396   Standard and Matrix, subsequent activities in LTTA 2 focused on the refinement of
397   these resources and further development of the EPICC Adoption Toolkit. Following
398   several rounds of intensive discussions between stakeholders, the nine competencies of
399   the draft EPICC Standard underwent significant revision to four competencies, with
400   outlined knowledge, skills and attitudes for each competence. Each of these competen-
401   cies is outlined in Chap. 1 and discussed further in Chaps. 5–8, respectively. The final
402   content and formatting of the EPICC Standard and Matrix was agreed at LTTA 2 and
403   approved by stakeholders at the final project event (ME 2). The EPICC Standard cap-
404   tures the complexity of the many competency items from Dr. Attard's PhD research,
405   whilst honouring the complex consensus method adopted by the project. The four com-
406   petencies are framed in the broader context of four 'themes': (1) intrapersonal spiritual-
407   ity; (2) interpersonal spirituality; (3) spiritual care: assessment and planning; and (4)
408   spiritual care: intervention and evaluation. This innovative approach helps to ensure
409   that the EPICC Standard has utility both in clinical practice by following the nursing/
410   midwifery processes, and in nursing/midwifery education by building knowledge,
411   skills, and attitudes incrementally across professional training.

When considering the EPICC Standard, it should not go unnoticed that this   412
was one of several resources produced during the project. Whilst the EPICC   413
Standard is arguably the most significant resource in helping to measure the   414
spiritual care competency of preregistration nurses/midwives, it is considered 415
to be one of the final aspects of professional development in spiritual care   416
before the point of professional registration. This process is illustrated through 417
the EPICC Matrix. During the latter part of LTTA 2, the EPICC Matrix under-   418
went significant refinement in respect of its content and presentation. This   419
EPICC Matrix is innovative in how it has utilised the key findings and recom- 420
mendations from 11 peer-reviewed studies in spiritual care to illustrate what is 421
known about students upon entering their programme of study, and the impor-   422
tance of the cultural, social, and political environment in which spiritual care 423
competency develops. The way in which preregistration nursing/midwifery   424
students are selected for professional training is an important consideration, 425
and students can be selected on more personal and value-based assessment in   426
addition to their grades. For example, in the UK, 'values-based recruitment' is 427
an important aspect in determining the personal as well as academic specifica- 428
tion of nursing/midwifery candidates; with honesty/trustworthiness, communi- 429
cation skills, sensitivity and compassion amongst other attributes being   430
important [26]. The EPICC Matrix acknowledges this complexity by providing   431
reference to some key areas, which research shows can predict spiritual care   432
competency development: compassion, caring, empathy, warmth, personal   433
spirituality, and one's view of spirituality and spiritual care. Since spiritual 434
care competency does not develop in isolation, but rather in a complex and   435
dynamic environment, the stakeholders from midwifery coined the colloquial   436
phrase: the 'amniotic sac' to highlight that. This is akin to the amniotic sac of 437
fluid inside the female uterus where the unborn baby develops and grows. This 438
professional development of spiritual care competency is illustrated on the   439
EPICC Matrix by means of (1) the teaching and learning environment, (2) the   440
student as a person, and (3) the clinical environment. The collection of 11 peer- 441
reviewed studies each offer empirical support for these various 'environments' 442
in which spiritual care competency is understood to develop. We hope that dur- 443
ing the time of professional training, the four-item EPICC Standard will be   444
referred to in order to appraise competency development. During the refine-   445
ment of the EPICC Matrix, the Strategic Partners and Project Manager consid-   446
ered that it would be essential to have an accompanying narrative for the EPICC 447
Matrix. This aims to help readers navigate the complexities of student selec- 448
tion, the environment in which spiritual care competency develops, and how   449
students are assessed to be competent in spiritual care at the point of profes- 450
sional registration. The Matrix narrative provides specific details for each of 451
the sections of the Matrix, but emphasises particular attention on the three   452
'environments', with detail from the literature.   453

9.4   Coronavirus Disease 2019 (COVID-19) and Spiritual Disruption?

We cannot conclude this chapter and indeed book without making any reference to COVID-19. The world is currently in the grip of a pandemic caused by the severe acute respiratory syndrome novel coronavirus 2 (SARS-CoV-2) resulting in COVID-19. The virus was first detected in Wuhan City, China, in December 2019. The virus once reported spread rapidly globally becoming a pandemic, which has had a devastating impact on the normal functioning of everyday life. It has placed tremendous strain on health and social care systems, halted economies, and has had a significant impact on people's lives, relationships, and activities. The response of governments has been unprecedented, costing billions to save lives, reduce the impact on hospital services, whilst preserving employment, and education. The World Health Organisation [27] reports that globally, as of 4 November 2020 (09:58), there have been 47,059,867 confirmed cases of COVID-19, including 1,207,327 deaths, reported to WHO. The rapid spread of COVID-19 across many countries has led to an international public health emergency and raised awareness of how countries monitor, prevent, and control the spread of the virus.

The World Health Organization declared 2020 as the International Year of the Nurse and Midwife. The importance and contribution of nurses and midwives has never been more important. Our societies have been affected by this virus causing a pandemic of unimaginable, almost apocalyptic proportions. The virus has disrupted and devastated every sphere of people's lives and existence. The virus has so far resulted in over one million deaths globally with many countries experiencing very high mortality rates. Furthermore, the effects of so-called 'long covid' are also yet to be well determined or understood, and the potential future challenges of people requiring on-going care and support (both physiologically, psychologically, *and one might imagine spiritually*) should not be underestimated [28]. The virus has also had a massive impact on the economic and financial infrastructures of many nations, with individuals not being able to work, many losing their jobs and livelihoods. Children and young people have been unable to attend school or educational institutions and family members and friends have had to isolate from each other during 'lockdowns.' Civil liberties have had to be curtailed and individuals have had to embrace and endure a wide range of measures that have restricted freedom and everyday living.

The virus has been indiscriminate, traversing all age and ethnic groups but has been particularly devasting to some vulnerable and at-risk groups, such as older people, those receiving treatment for conditions such as cancer, and those living with long-term conditions. The human suffering has been immense, but this has been compounded by all the restrictions that have had to be imposed to control the rate and spread of the virus. Nursing, midwifery, and healthcare have been at the frontline of the pandemic having to care for some very seriously ill individuals who have required considerable critical and life-saving care in high-dependency and critical care units.

When one looks at the impact of the COVID-19 pandemic, the importance of the spiritual dimension of people's lives becomes very clear. As the many definitions of spirituality presented throughout this book affirm, the concept concerns those important aspects of people's lives which might be taken for granted. For example, what can be deemed the ordinary and mundane activities of everyday life; our relationships, employment, recreation, being able to practice one's religion, and ultimately offering support to loved ones who are experiencing illness and approaching the end of life. It is not until the ordinary and mundane things we take for granted are threatened or removed, that we appreciate the significance and value we place upon them and the important structural role they play in our lives. The fundamental attributes of spirituality: meaning, purpose and fulfilment (existential), transcendence, religiosity, relationships and connections have all been affected, meaning that many individuals are experiencing what could be termed a 'spiritual disruption' to everyday existence.

The 'spiritual disruption' caused by the COVID-19 pandemic has been unprecedented, because every sphere and aspect of people's lives have been devastated and almost dismantled. There has been a shattering of everything that can be deemed normal. Yet, during what could be considered a very bleak and traumatic time, we have witnessed the best of humanity and communities rallying to support each other and especially the most vulnerable. There have been heroic accounts of individuals, nurses, midwives, and healthcare professionals going above and beyond, in the face of great adversity to ensure those affected by COVID-19 receive compassionate care. New and innovative ways of maintaining connections between family members across many sectors of health and social care have had to be created, especially for those receiving palliative and end-of-life care.

Nurses and midwives throughout this pandemic have shown considerable courage and resilience, drawing on their own spiritual resources to ensure those in need of care feel respected and valued. Yet, the demands on nurses and midwives have been visible, with many having to spend considerable time working under extreme pressures and conditions, wearing personal and protective equipment for long hours, and dealing with situations that are very emotionally and psychologically distressing. The moral injury and spiritual distress caused by the pandemic on those working in frontline services is still to manifest. The long-term cost, impact and ramifications of the pandemic upon individuals, our nursing, midwifery, and healthcare professions will be significant. The importance of spirituality will play an important part in the recovery and healing both individually and across societies.

9.5 The Future

The EPICC Network was launched on 2 July 2019 and presently has 77 members. The network has members in most continents including Europe, Asia, Africa and Australia. The network exists to promote evidence-based spiritual care education and practice across Europe and beyond, and aims to bring together experts in the field and those who are new to this area. The network is for those interested in developing nursing/midwifery spiritual care education and practice.

The EPICC website has been updated so that this can support the advancement of the network, particularly in respect of communications between the network members and the public. The former EPICC project website has been updated reflecting the transition from the project to the much wider EPICC Network. All outputs from the former EPICC project have been archived on the updated website. The main goal of the new website is to inform network members about developments, publications and events about spiritual care education in nursing and midwifery. It will also act as a repository by signposting visitors to recent publications that have used the EPICC project outputs in their research or work.

References

1. Nursing and Midwifery Council (NMC). Standards of competence for registered nurses. 2010. https://www.nmc.org.uk/globalassets/sitedocuments/standards/nmc-standards-for-competence-for-registered-nurses.pdf. Accessed 22 Oct 2020.
2. Nursing and Midwifery Council (NMC). Future nurse: Standards of proficiency for registered nurses. 2018. https://www.nmc.org.uk/globalassets/sitedocuments/education-standards/future-nurse-proficiencies.pdf. Accessed 22 Oct 2020.
3. Nursing and Midwifery Council (NMC). Standards of proficiency for midwives. 2019. https://www.nmc.org.uk/globalassets/sitedocuments/standards/standards-of-proficiency-for-midwives.pdf. Accessed 24 Oct 2020.
4. Rushton L. What are the barriers to spiritual care in a hospital setting? Br J Nurs. 2014;23:370–4. https://doi.org/10.12968/bjon.2014.23.7.370.
5. Ross L. Spiritual care in nursing: an overview of the research to date. J Clin Nurs. 2006;15:852–62. https://doi.org/10.1111/j.1365-2702.2006.01617.x.
6. Narayanasamy A. Nurses' awareness and educational preparation in meeting their patients' spiritual needs. Nurse Educ Today. 1993;13:196–201. https://doi.org/10.1016/0260-6917(93)90102-8.
7. Ross L. Teaching spiritual care to nurses. Nurse Educ Today. 1996;16:38–43. https://doi.org/10.1016/S0260-6917(96)80091-8.
8. van Leeuwen R, Cusveller B. Nursing competencies for spiritual care. J Adv Nurs. 2004;48:234–46. https://doi.org/10.1111/j.1365-2648.2004.03192.x.
9. Cockell N, McSherry W. Spiritual care in nursing: an overview of published international research. J Nurs Manag. 2012;20:958–69. https://doi.org/10.1111/j.1365-2834.2012.01450.x.
10. de Souza JR, Maftum MA, de Azevedo Mazza V. The nursing care in the spiritual dimension: undergraduates' experience. Online Braz J Nurs. 2009;12:743–5. https://doi.org/10.5935/1676-4285.20092127.
11. van Leeuwen R, Tiesinga LJ, Middel B, Post D, Jochemsen H. The effectiveness of an educational programme for nursing students on developing competence in the provision of spiritual care. J Clin Nurs. 2008;17:2768–81. https://doi.org/10.1111/j.1365-2702.2008.02366.x.
12. van Leeuwen R, Tiesinga LJ, Middel B, Post D, Jochemsen H. The validity and reliability of an instrument to assess nursing competencies in spiritual care. J Clin Nurs. 2009;18:2857–969. https://doi.org/10.1111/j.1365-2702.2008.02594.x.
13. Ross L, van Leeuwen R, Baldacchino D, Giske T, McSherry W, Narayanasamy A, Downes C, Jarvis P, Schep-Akkerman A. Student nurses perceptions of spirituality and competence in delivering spiritual care: a European pilot study. Nurse Educ Today. 2014;34:697–702. https://doi.org/10.1016/j.nedt.2013.09.014.
14. Ross L, Giske T, van Leeuwen R, Baldacchino D, McSherry W, Narayanasamy A, Downs C, Jarvis P, Schep-Akkerman A. Factors contributing to student nurses'/midwives' per-

ceived competence in spiritual care: findings from a European pilot study. Nurse Educ Today. 2016;36:445–51. https://doi.org/10.1016/j.nedt.2015.10.005.

15. Ross L, McSherry W, Giske T, van Leeuwen R, Schep-Akkerman A, Koslander T, Hall J, Steenfeldt VØ, Jarvis P. Nursing and midwifery students' perceptions of spirituality, spiritual care, and spiritual care competency: a prospective, longitudinal, correlational European study. Nurse Educ Today. 2018;67:64–71. https://doi.org/10.1016/j.nedt.2018.05.002.

16. Giske T, Cone PH. Opening up to learning spiritual care of patients: a grounded theory study of nursing students. J Clin Nurs. 2012;21:2006–15. https://doi.org/10.1111/j.1365-2702.2011.04054.x.

17. Kuven B, Giske T. Talking about spiritual matters: first years nursing students' experiences of an assignment on spiritual care conversation. Nurse Educ Today. 2019;75:53–7. https://doi.org/10.1016/j.nedt.2019.01.012.

18. Royal College of Nursing (RCN). RCN spirituality survey 2010. 2011. https://www.rcn.org.uk/professional-development/publications/pub-003861. Accessed 9 Apr 2019.

19. Revans R. ABC of action learning. Farnham: Gower; 2011.

20. Erasmus+. Glossary. n.d. https://www.erasmusplus.org.uk/glossary. Accessed 24 Oct 2020.

21. Royal College of Nursing (RCN). RCN ViPERS guidelines for session facilitators: What is a ViPER? 2019. https://www.rcn.org.uk/-/media/royal-college-of-nursing/documents/events/2019/september/research-2019/viper-guidelines.pdf?la=en&hash=CF4ADB3153245A431E7A16E2F8970BD879ADEFC1. Accessed 24 Oct 2020.

22. Chung LYF, Wong FKY, Chan MF. Relationship of nurses' spirituality to their understanding and practice of spiritual care. J Adv Nurs. 2007;58:158–70. https://doi.org/10.1111/j.1365-2648.2007.04225.x.

23. van Leeuwen R, Attard J, Ross L, Boughey A, Giske T, Kleiven T, McSherry W. The development of a consensus-based spiritual care education standard for undergraduate nursing and midwifery students. J Adv Nurs. 2020;77:973–86. https://doi.org/10.1111/jan.14613.

24. Attard J, Ross L, Weeks KW. Design and development of a spiritual care competency framework for pre-registration nurses and midwives: a modified Delphi study. Nurse Educ Pract. 2019;39:96–104. https://doi.org/10.1016/j.nepr.2019.08.003.

25. Attard J, Ross L, Weeks KW. Developing a spiritual care competency framework for pre-registration nurses and midwives. Nurse Educ Pract. 2019;40:102604. https://doi.org/10.1016/j.nepr.2019.07.010.

26. Waugh A, Smith D, Horsburgh D, Gray M. Towards a values-based person specification for recruitment of compassionate nursing and midwifery candidates: a study of registered and student nurses' and midwives' perceptions of prerequisite attributes and key skills. Nurse Educ Today. 2014;34:1190–5. https://doi.org/10.1016/j.nedt.2013.12.009.

27. World Health Organization (WHO). WHO Coronavirus Disease (COVID-19) Dashboard. 2020. https://covid19.who.int/. Accessed 4 Nov 2020.

28. Mahase E. Covid-19: what do we know about "long covid"? Br Med J. 2020;370:m2815. https://doi.org/10.1136/bmj.m2815.

Suggested Reading

McSherry W. Enhancing and advancing spiritual care in nursing and midwifery practice. Nursing Standard. 2020;35:65–8. https://doi.org/10.7748/ns.35.10.65.s35. https://journals.rcni.com/nursing-standard/feature/enhancing-and-advancing-spiritual-care-in-nursing-and-midwifery-practice-ns.35.10.65.s35/pdf. Accessed 4 Nov 2020.

van Leeuwen R, Attard J, Ross L, Boughey A, Giske T, Kleiven T, McSherry W. The development of a consensus-based spiritual care education standard for undergraduate nursing and mid-wifery students. J Adv Nurs. 2020;77:973–86. https://doi.org/10.1111/jan.14613.

Afterword: Compassion in Care

In some ways this book should not be necessary. As nurses and midwives, society might expect that we are compassionate and considerate of spirituality for all those within our care. However, it is evident from the degree of technology used within healthcare and the advances in robotic medicine that it lacks humanity. Indeed, if one were to read any hospital complaint records or sadly national reports into investigations of services, they would show that communication and deficits in compassion feature throughout.

Michel Foucault warned the medical world that objectifying the body under a 'medical gaze' creates a perfect system to dehumanise clinical care, where only the condition is of interest to the medical person. Healthcare over the past century has rapidly advanced, and the health of our societies has benefitted hugely. Nonetheless, the more sophisticated medicine has become, the greater the need for holistic care, so that the humanity of the person who may be ill or receiving care has all of their needs met.

In the foreword of this book, the author commented upon the care of the dying; this is an area of interest to me and was at the very heart of my thoughts when designing and articulating the vision of midwifery units that I have created. If we look at birth and death as a dyad, then it is impossible to separate these most critical of life events and not attending to the spirituality of the person is to omit an essential part of what makes us human. Indeed, when I was meeting with architects and designers in this stage of development for a Birth Centre, I asked the project manager to visit two hospices in our local area. I needed them to see and feel what was important in making death a compassionate experience for all involved including the staff who worked there. In the final plans and schedule of what was non-negotiable was the dimly lit rooms and corridors, the accessibility of refreshments when they were needed, the integration of bathrooms within each room so that dignity was maintained and the fact that a whole family could be with a woman when she was birthing and stay until they were ready for home. This design for Serenity Birth Centre was unique at the time but very soon became a national and international standard, a place that birth and the sanctity of that experience was nurtured.

© Springer Nature Switzerland AG 2021
W. McSherry et al. (eds.), *Enhancing Nurses' and Midwives' Competence in Providing Spiritual Care*, https://doi.org/10.1007/978-3-030-65888-5

32   Some might argue that you cannot teach spirituality and compassion, that it is an
33   individual trait that is within us and perhaps learnt as a child throughout our parent-
34   ing. However, that is not entirely true. Florence Nightingale taught her nurses that
35   'apprehension, uncertainty, waiting, expectation, fear of surprise, do a patient more
36   harm than any exertion'. Clearly, she was aware that out of our normal environ-
37   ments and suffering pain and discomfort would increase our distress which could be
38   soothed by a compassionate healer.

39   The authors in this book have made eloquent and complex advances for the
40   teaching and understanding of compassion within the academic teachings of nurs-
41   ing and midwifery. They argue that unless these elements are included within our
42   training, we risk becoming robotic and systematic rather than responsive and com-
43   passionate. The work that has gone into ensuring that spirituality is integrated into
44   learning is more than holistic rather it is inherent throughout the text. They have
45   attempted to direct others that this route is vital and should encourage all higher
46   institutes of academic teaching to adopt this approach. After all, compassion is not
47   a weakness, it is a strength that holds the patient in the moment we are with them.

48   It is not easy in our modern multicultural society to try to understand and adopt
49   typologies that reflect the breadth of cultural and religious needs of all of us. In fact,
50   I would argue that it is impossible. However, that has not been denied by the authors,
51   they have embraced individualism and the sanctity of the 'person'. The one to one-
52   ness of being with someone who may be fearful of their pain and how they might
53   cope can be moderated by a caring nurse/midwife who reaches out to them compas-
54   sionately and is there by their side. This is the nub of the book. Being with, entirely
55   focussed on, speaking quietly with love and care, listening to what the patient/
56   woman says and knowing sometimes that words are not necessary. I believe that any
57   training or learning that upholds these qualities has to improve our healthcare sys-
58   tems and more than this will benefit not only the patient but the carer.

59   I fully endorse this book and its intention to treat the human within our caring.
60   Teaching how to care in practice is fully achievable—so it is now vital that we find
61   ways to articulate and reach the spiritual part of our patients'/families' needs. It may
62   be uncomfortable at times; it may challenge those of us who struggle to find our own
63   spirituality, but then if we have made such advances in science and medicine, then
64   this should be possible. As nurses and midwives, we have chosen a path to be with
65   the sick and birthing families; we have dedicated our clinical practice to do no harm.
66   Let us now commit to fulfilling the spiritual and humanity of those in our care. It will
67   give us increased satisfaction in our work and draw us closer to those we tend.

68   I hope that as reader you will enjoy this book but more than that will be a pioneer
69   of compassion and love for the human side of what we do in nursing and midwifery.

70   Michel Foucault. The Birth of the Clinic: An Archaeology of Medical Perception.
71   (Naissance de la clinique: une archéologie du regard médical, 1963).

72   Royal College of Midwives, London, UK   Kathryn Gutteridge

Author Queries

Chapter No.: 0005083973

Queries	Details Required	Author's Response
AU1	Please clarify whether "foreword" could be changed to "preface".	
AU2	Rather than 'none negotiable', should this be 'non-negotiable?	